T0270922

Women's Sexual and Reproductive Health

Women's Sexual and Reproductive Health addresses the sexual and reproductive health needs of Asian American, Native Hawaiian, and Pacific Islander (AANHPI) women from a structural and intersectional perspective.

AANHPI women in the United States have often been grouped together due to their race and gender, regardless of their specific communities' diverse histories with the United States and different educational and economic opportunities. The authors argue that AANHPI women are misunderstood by health professionals and researchers, and foregrounds AANHPI women's experiences to demonstrate the challenges they face when seeking health care. The book highlights the diversity of AANHPI women by drawing on their first-hand experiences, and argues for the disaggregation of health data on AANHPI women.

Women's Sexual and Reproductive Health is of value to college classrooms that address racial disparities, health disparities, and women's experiences, as well as for health care professionals.

Karen J. Leong is Associate Professor of History at University of New Mexico. Her research explores what Asian American experiences reveal about the historical dynamic between U.S. national ideologies and the power of self-definition at the intersections of gender, race, class, and sexuality.

Kathy Nakagawa is Associate Professor Emeritus of Asian Pacific American studies in the School of Social Transformation at Arizona State University. Her research explores issues of inequity in education including the relationship between families and schools, parent involvement and school reform, charter schools, family literacy programs and racial literacy.

Aggie J. Yellow Horse is Associate Professor of Asian Pacific American Studies in the School of Social Transformation at Arizona State University. Her research focuses on understanding how larger social forces "get under the skin" to generate health inequities for racialized and minoritized peoples.

Routledge Focus on Gender, Sexuality & Praxis

Women's Sexual and Reproductive Health
Visibility, Equality, and AANHPI
Karen J. Leong, Kathy Nakagawa, and Aggie J. Yellow Horse

For more information about this series, please visit: https://www.routledge.com/Routledge-Focus-on-Gender-Sexuality-and-Praxis/book-series/FGSP

Women's Sexual and Reproductive Health

Recognition, Equity, and AANHPI

Karen J. Leong,
Kathy Nakagawa, and
Aggie J. Yellow Horse

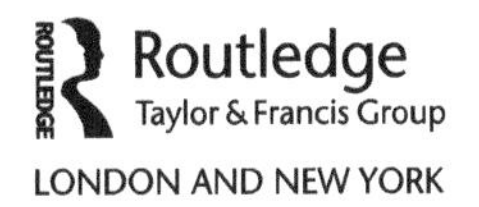

LONDON AND NEW YORK

First published 2024
by Routledge
4 Park Square, Milton Park, Abingdon, Oxon OX14 4RN

and by Routledge
605 Third Avenue, New York, NY 10158

Routledge is an imprint of the Taylor & Francis Group, an informa business

British Library Cataloguing-in-Publication Data
A catalogue record for this book is available from the British Library

ISBN: 978-1-032-58386-0 (hbk)
ISBN: 978-1-032-58389-1 (pbk)
ISBN: 978-1-003-44986-7 (ebk)

DOI: 10.4324/9781003449867

Typeset in Times New Roman
by MPS Limited, Dehradun

Contents

Acknowledgements

The authors acknowledge that this collaborative work would not have been possible without each other. In 2018, Aggie Yellow Horse initiated this collaboration and under her leadership we secured funding for a research project that resulted in The Arizona Asian American and Pacific Islander Women's Health Project. We thank our community partners and community members who worked with us to make this project a reality: Claudia Kaercher and Island Liaison LLC, Arizona Matsuri: Festival of Japan, Arizona Aloha Festival, Asian Pacific Community in Action, Planned Parenthood Arizona. We are indebted to performance artist Kristina Wong who generously collaborated with us (and our shoestring budget) for the public event, and facilitated a humorous, engaging, and reflective discussion among the community participants about AANHPI women's sexual and reproductive health. A seed grant from Arizona State University's Institute of Humanities Research provided funding for the project, and we appreciate our colleagues who as IHR Health Humanities fellows provided their insights and knowledge as we developed the project.

We are grateful to H.L.T. Quan, editor of the FOCUS book series, for suggesting and believing in this book as well as guiding us through the book proposal process. We thank Jodie Collins, editorial assistant for Taylor & Francis and the book series for her support and guidance. We thank the anonymous manuscript reviewers for their generative feedback for the manuscript, and Astha Rohit who as an ASU undergraduate student also provided her valuable critique of the manuscript and helped to identify community organizations for the appendix.

Introduction

When Mitsuye Yamada, a Japanese American poet and activist for women's rights, observed that "Invisibility is an unnatural disaster," she was addressing the invisibility of Asian American women in U.S. society and the costs of that invisibility for women. "One of the most insidious ways of keeping women and minorities powerless," she wrote, "is to let them only talk about harmless and inconsequential subjects or let them speak freely and not listen to them with serious intent" (Yamada, 1979, p. 40). This book is about Asian American, Native Hawaiian, and Pacific Islander women's sexual and reproductive[1] health and confronts the ongoing inattention to these women's perspectives about sexual health in research, practice, and policy (Wang Kong et al., 2022). We use the term Asian American, Native Hawaiian, and Pacific Islander (AANHPI hereafter) specifically to disaggregate the historical legacies of these communities (discussed in chapter 1) that have historically been grouped together indiscriminately by the U.S. government in data collection such as the federal census.[2] While we use U.S. terminology as published in the Census and other documents, we also use the punctuation and terminology preferred by Indigenous Pacific Islanders to refer to themselves and their nations. This includes American Sāmoa, Sāmoa, and Sāmoan, Guåhan (instead of Guam), CHamoru (instead of Chamorro), Hawai`i, and Kānaka Maoli interchangeably with Native Hawaiians.

The lack of attention to AANHPI women's health relates to a combination of societal factors. How does this lack of research and knowledge about cultural and other factors among medical practitioners affect AANHPI women's health and their willingness to address their sexual health with their health care providers? Community norms and personal circumstances may further inform whether individual women feel empowered to advocate for their own health care. Although Chou's (2012) important work has addressed the norms of race, gender, and sexuality in Asian ethnic communities and U.S. whitestream society that differentiate social expectations for Asian American men and women,

DOI: 10.4324/9781003449867-1

her work does not focus on health specifically. Research that does highlight AANHPI women's health tends to focus on mental health rather than their sexual and reproductive health.[3] In this book, we attempt to address the complex combination of social factors and specific personal circumstances that contribute to neglect regarding AANHPI women's sexual and reproductive health. Sexual and reproductive health are part of AANHPI women's experiences, and we can address the broader issues relating to sexual and reproductive health without the reticence and shame that often accompany these discussions.

> I remember my mom saying, "You don't have sex until you are married," and that whole, "Don't have sex 'til you're married, don't ever" ... And then I thought she'd only had sex with my Dad. Like I never knew there was any life prior to or after. ... I later learned like she was having an affair, and she had an abortion when she was younger ... And I didn't know that 'til somebody else told me. ... and I think it has a lot to do with the shame, and the expectation that you need to be perfect, you need to present to the community that everything is great in our house. ... And it's funny because thinking about that and how it effects my health, there is that expectation in my mind that whatever you do has to be great, don't bring shame. That stress of trying to be perfect, and trying to build this person of "Everything is great in my life," even though my health may be falling apart.
>
> *-Kasey,*[4] *Focus group participant*

Just as Kasey noted, too often the topics of sex and reproduction are taboo. Furthermore, health care as a social institution also reflects the racism, sexism, homophobia and transphobia, classism, ableism, and other value systems embedded in our society. These systems work together not only to negatively affect AANHPI women's health but also to discourage us from seeking preventative health care. These systems may also work together to create conditions in which we think our health is not a priority in relation to other demands. Work, childcare, and housework frequently are expected of women in the U.S. Caring for elders, contributing labor to community institutions, and sustaining social networks across extended kin and community often are also part of the invisible labor of AANHPI women in their communities. For example, some AANHPI cultures assume that the mother feeds everyone else first before herself. These gendered expectations, along with sexual and reproductive health, often are not openly addressed nor discussed – much to the detriment of AANHPI women's quality of life.

At the same time, it is dangerous to generalize that AANHPI women share the same experiences. Those value systems that create familiar conditions for AANHPI women in relation to society also differentiate among AANHPI women. Moreover, AANHPI experiences vary based on one's specific culture (which is not simply nation-based but may reflect religious affiliation, class, language and/or caste status in that culture), immigrant generation, as well as one's specific legal status in relation to the United States (whether one is a citizen of a U.S. territory, a permanent resident, or on a work visa, and so forth). Given the vast differences among AANHPIs, even community members make assumptions about other ethnicities and their histories and experiences. This book thus seeks to demystify sexual and reproductive health among AANHPI women as well as the assumption of shared experiences among Asian American women or Native Hawaiians and Pacific Islander women on the basis of race. This educational goal is meant to empower AANHPI community members and communities collectively to better advocate for more effective and culturally responsive health care for AANHPI women. We also draw upon the work of feminist-of-color disability studies scholars who argue for "a critical and expansive approach to health/care," and "taking into account cultural and religious perspectives on wellness and healing, which may run counter to … Western white medical perspectives on these issues" (Schalk & Kim, 2020, p. 46).

This educational goal is also why we have chosen to address Native Hawaiian and Pacific Islander women's experiences alongside Asian American experiences in this book. Our own experiences as Asian American women living in Arizona have shown us that generalizing AANHPI experiences from data gathered on similar populations in large metropolitan communities such as those in California, New York, Texas, New Jersey, Washington, Nevada, or Utah, or the concentrations of Asian American or Native Hawaiian and Pacific Islander communities in Hawai'i or California, for example, can be misleading and distort the lived realities of smaller, often overlooked AANHPI communities. Although significant reasons exist for Native Hawaiian and Pacific Islanders to seek disaggregation from Asian Americans and even from each other (as will be discussed in Chapter 1), some communities have found reason to work together in order to access local and state attention and resources. For example, the relatively smaller numbers of Asian Americans, Native Hawaiians, and Pacific Islanders in Arizona concentrated in three counties – Maricopa, Pima and Cochise – has resulted in interaction and collaboration over the years. When Asian Pacific American Studies first began as a certificate at Arizona State University in 1998, Pacific Islander community leaders specifically asked that "Pacific" be included in the name of the program because they had participated in the discussions and advocacy for such a program for over twenty years.

Today, many pan-ethnic organizations such as Asian Pacific Community in Action, Pan Asian Community Alliance and Arizona Asian Americans, Native Hawaiians and Pacific Islanders for Equity represent the contributions of and serve Asian Americans, Native Hawaiians, and Pacific Islanders. Even long-time community groups such as the Japanese American Citizens League, Arizona Chapter work with other organizations to serve the broader AANHPI community. This collaboration was evident in the community-based research that inspired this book – equal numbers of Pacific Islanders and Asian Americans participated in our study, due in large part to the support of Island Liaison, LLC, a non-profit organization in Arizona that has advocated for Pacific Islander education, health, and culture since 2012. However, although we demonstrate the distinct histories of Pacific Islanders from Asian Americans in Chapter 1, due to the small numbers of Pacific Islanders in the Phoenix Metropolitan area, we do not identify the ethnicity of the focus group participant for specific quotes throughout the book in order to protect identities.

The firsthand experiences that we highlight in this book have a context that is specific to our location. Nonetheless, we believe that these experiences also speak to larger historical, cultural and social patterns that frame the ways in which AANHPI women have been perceived and understood in U.S. society, including by health care providers. And this has important consequences for the health and well-being of AANHPI women at large.

> I'm just wondering when growing up when we thought of health it was more illness. Sickness … . Whereas as I got older and wiser, I learned health to be wellness. Balance. … again, how do you wrap yourself around this health stuff?
>
> *-Fran, Focus group participant*

We envisioned this book as having multiple access points. The introduction begins the conversation about AANHPI women's sexual and reproductive health by defining terms. In this introduction, we focus on what we mean by health overall and sexual and reproductive health. We then highlight the ways AANHPI women are overlooked by providing an overview of why and how AANHPI women are understudied in health equity and policy research. For those who would like to learn more about the histories of AANHPI communities and how literature, poetry and other media inform the study of AANHPI women's health experiences, Chapter 1 provides this focus. Understanding the specific relationships Asian Americans, Native Hawaiians, and Pacific Islanders have had with the United States is vital to understanding their diverse yet related experiences in the U.S. context and helps to illuminate health disparities and access to health care. The chapter identifies key characteristics of the United States' AANHPI population and explores how Asian Americans and Pacific Islanders' vast range of experiences in the United States are nonetheless distilled into popular stereotypes about AANHPI women through media and policy. Using literature and poetry, we examine how these stereotypes may inform misleading assumptions about AANHPI women's knowledge about and comfort with discussing sexual and reproductive health. These stereotypes in fact, may undermine attention to the whole of AANHPI women's lived experiences, which need to be accounted for in addressing their health. All of this context is critical, because "when education is culturally specific and tailored to the unique issues and needs of the targeted community, it is more likely to lead to positive outcomes. … Effectiveness is enhanced because culturally specific interventions are more likely to attract targeted participants" (Robinson et al., 2002, p. 46).

Readers who may be more familiar with history but are less knowledgeable about issues related to AANHPI data and the importance of data disaggregation for understanding the diversity of AANHPIs may want to delve into Chapter 2. In Chapter 2, we focus on one important aspect of the systemic challenges to understanding AANHPI women's overall health including sexual and reproductive health – namely, challenges in representation in data and methods in "scientific" research. We discuss the importance of adequate and just representation of AANHPIs in data and the need for meaningful data disaggregation for AANHPI communities by illustrating how the common practice of data aggregation can mask the important and diverse sexual and reproductive health profiles, desires and needs among highly diverse AANHPI women. In order for individuals and communities to better advocate for themselves, we believe that data literacy is vital. Certain types of data are used to determine health treatment and public health policy, yet lumping together AANHPI health data may result in specific health risks and behaviors being misrepresented and ignored.

Those who are interested in hearing specific voices of AANHPI women and some of the ways we gathered stories and began having conversations about sexual and reproductive health may want to start with Chapter 3. Chapter 3 illustrates how utilizing storytelling as a means of data gathering allows access to the diversity of lived experiences and perspectives essential to understanding AANHPI women's health. Drawing on the *Arizona Asian American and Pacific Islander Women's Health Project* (more details later), the chapter includes some of the ways the participants in the project discussed their own sexual and reproductive health, and how the sense of community space and support as well as the storytelling process were important for individual empowerment and community building. We also include some of the ways the storytelling opened up the research project to new modes of research and presentation.

The book concludes with Chapter 4, which provides specific activities for researchers, community organizations, and health care providers to create spaces for understanding the diversity of the AANHPI women's sexual and reproductive health experiences. The activities are meant to provide support for individuals and groups to enter into conversations that ensure they are heard with "serious intent."

The book has two appendices. Appendix B provides a list of national AANHPI organizations that provide relevant resources that may be of interest to readers seeking to learn more or develop their own community organizations. Appendix A provides the survey and focus group script we used for the Arizona Asian American Pacific Islander Women's Health Project.

Conceptualizing Health: Individualization of Health vs. Population Health

Before we think about how we measure health in data, it is important to have conversations about how we think about and conceptualize health. In 1948, the World Health Organization (WHO) constituted the definition of health as "a state of complete physical, mental and social well-being and not merely the absence of disease or infirmity" (WHO, 2002). Health often is conceptualized as an individual matter as heavily influenced by the medical perspective. Indeed, individuals experience health and health changes in their own bodies, and it is a critical and private matter for individuals. However, WHO's very definition of health refutes the notion that health is only an individual matter by its emphasis on its social aspects (e.g., an individual's ability to interact and have meaningful relationships with others). In other words, health also can be understood as "a state of balance within oneself and with the environment" (Sartorius, 2006, p. 662). In a broad sense, a person's health is not only defined by one's individual health and health behaviors, but also is greatly influenced by one's surroundings – how healthy are one's loved ones in the family and community. As Yuri Kochiyama (2004) observed, "Life is not what you alone make it. Life is the input of everyone who touched your life and every experience that entered it. We are all part of one another" (Kochiyama et al., 2004). In other words, individuals do not exist in isolation but in relationships. Our health also does not exist in isolation, but in relation to one another. This is particularly important when considering AANHPI women's health.

This point almost appears common sense and innate given our own lived experiences; but highlighting such a notion has important implications about how we think about health about ourselves, our family, and our community. The notion of "individualization of health" (Mendenhall, 2016), prominent in medicine, solely focuses on individual characteristics to understand health. This approach puts great emphasis on individuals' health status and health behaviors (e.g., eating a healthy diet and exercise), and puts the responsibility of health solely on individuals. This approach becomes highly problematic as it does not account for larger social conditions (e.g., social and physical environments, social relationships, etc.) that can affect individuals above and beyond their personal characteristics. This translates to the importance of understanding the "social determinants of health."

The social determinants of health refer to the social conditions in which people are born, grow, live and work; they are considered the mechanisms of fundamental causes of health (Link & Phelan, 1995; Phelan et al., 2010). This means that while individual factors such as diet and exercise are important proximal factors that influence health, they are simply the mechanisms of how the social conditions translate to different health status and outcomes. For example, not using any birth control contraceptive methods (an individual's health behavior) can lead to a mistimed or unintended pregnancy (an individual's health outcome). Yet, a woman might not have used any birth control contraceptives because she does not have access to a health insurance, have transportation to get to the doctor's office, or is unable to pay for the prescription – all of which reflect the social circumstances of her life. These social circumstances may reflect institutional decisions beyond an individual's control on the part of whether an employer provides health insurance coverage or whether a local government invests in public transportation, or whether individuals living with disabilities have access to accommodations. Each of the chapters in this book offers different ways of moving beyond individualization of health when considering AANHPI women's sexual and reproductive health.

Another way to move beyond the "individualization of health" is to think about the health of the population. Population health is defined as "the health outcomes of a group of individuals, including the distribution of such outcomes within the group" (Kindig & Stoddart, 2003, p. 380). Population can be defined at multiple geographic scales – e.g., AANHPI women in Phoenix (city), AANHPI women in Arizona (state), AANHPI women in the United States (national), etc. Conceptualizing health as a group – collective health – is critical as it provides "an opportunity for health care systems, agencies and organizations to work together in order to improve the health outcomes of the communities they serve" (CFPH., 2020). Population health research can lead to improved access to care and better patient engagement for the community. Public health policies often use population health research to allocate funding to reduce and eliminate health inequities – the unjust and unfair distribution of health resources, outcomes, and determinants across groups (Braveman & Gottlieb, 2014). Therefore, being able to critically assess and understand the community's health is directly related to how effectively we can advocate for more institutional support for promoting the health of our community (Kindig & Stoddart, 2003; Lantz et al., 2007). Communities so often are defined by those who represent the majority of its members, and this may result in overlooking the specificities of those whose bodies, health, sexual orientation, ethnicity, citizenship, class status, disability, or other characteristics do not represent those of the majority. Conceptualizing health as a simultaneously individual and collective matter, this book concludes with a chapter that considers next steps for promoting AANHPI community health.

What Is Sexual and Reproductive Health?

Sexual and reproductive health may be an unfamiliar idea. While the dictionary defines health as being "1 a: the condition of being sound in body, mind, or spirit; *especially*: free from physical disease or pain," (Merriam-Webster.com, 2023) and one's physical sex refers to the parts of the body involved in biological reproduction (such as the penis, uterus, vulva, and testicles), one's sexuality is not simply biological. One's sexuality may also refer to physical pleasure in which case some have argued that the human skin may be the largest human sexual organ. However, sexuality is not simply biological nor physical. Sexuality includes emotional attraction towards other people. One may be emotionally or physically attracted to someone of the opposite sex (heterosexual), the same sex (homosexual), any sex (pansexual), or experience little or no attraction at all (asexual). Similarly, health encompasses much more than one's physical body. The World Health Organization defines sexual health as "the state of physical, emotional, mental, and social well-being in relation to sexuality" (WHO, 2006, p. 5). This means that any discussion of sexual health must take into account the multiple factors – physical, mental, emotional, social, and/or spiritual – that affect an individual and their intimate relationships with others (Hillman, 2011; Lindau et al., 2003). This more comprehensive understanding of sexual well-being also assumes that one's sexual health is connected to one's overall well-being, and that one's sexuality is intimately connected to one's self-knowledge and self-perception. To feel confident about their sexual needs and wants and to be able to clearly communicate those to a sexual partner, individuals should feel at ease with who they are and know what they find comfortable and safe. They also must be able to communicate concerns and questions with their health care provider.

Key aspects of sexual health include (Edwards & Coleman, 2004; Robinson et al., 2002):

- Self-awareness and acceptance of one's values, attitudes, and behaviors
- Accurate and appropriate knowledge about one's body and sexual functions
- Communicative about needs and desires relating to sex and intimacy

- Awareness of any life challenges to one's sexual health and satisfaction
- Freedom to act and freedom from coercion and abuse
- Understanding cultural definitions of what constitutes pleasure and desire

Just as individuals are encouraged to be aware and comfortable about their bodies, desire, and pleasure in order to communicate with their intimate partners, the ability to communicate about their bodies and assert their health needs is vital in working with the health care system. The health care system often does not allot time for conversations to build trust or understanding, even if a patient may have a preferred provider. Health care providers, while trained to address physical issues, may not be trained to address the range of differences that inform how individuals relate to their own bodies. Cultural competency is almost always generalized, and it is important that individuals feel comfortable correcting any assumptions made on the basis of perceived racial or cultural identity. Developing confidence in communicating one's needs is a process that begins with learning how one's own values, beliefs, and circumstances affect one's sexual health and overall sense of well-being. Understanding this relationship between well-being and health and social systems is the basis of reproductive justice.

Reproductive justice advocates equity in reproductive health – holistic health and well-being in all matters relating to the reproductive system and to its functions and processes, and "the freedom to decide if, when and how often to do so" (WHO, 2002). The Reproductive Justice movement began in 1994 among twelve Black women in Chicago, who formed Women of African Descent for Reproductive Justice (WADRJ) and demanded that any health care reforms pay attention to Black women's needs, which included racial and economic disparities (Abrams, 2019; Ross et al., 2016). In 1997, a coalition of Black, Latinx, Indigenous and Asian American women created SisterSong collective to promote the sexual and reproductive health of women of color and gender expansive people of color (Ross et al., 2016). Loretta Ross, one of the original twelve women who formed WADRJ, quotes Asian Communities for Reproductive Justice, "Reproductive Justice is the complete physical, mental, spiritual, political, social, and economic well-being of women and girls, based in the full achievement and protection of women's human rights" (Abrams, 2019). This movement embraces social justice in demanding a healthy environment, and basic human rights of shelter, food and health (care) for all people regardless of gender, sexual orientation, race, disability, or citizenship status. Regardless of whether a person chooses to give birth to a child or not, parent or not, the focus is on building communities that support health and well-being (Ross, 2007).

Maria Nakae of Asian Communities for Reproductive Justice (ACRJ) –one of the founding members of the SisterSong collective – emphasizes that AANHPI women also encounter economic and racial disparities. AANHPI immigrant women often are employed in low-wage jobs where they also may be exposed to toxic substances in their places of work. They may lack access to public assistance and social services because they lack U.S. citizenship. Nakae (2007) notes, "Every day, API women face challenges to their bodily self-determination" (p.16), including lack of access to information, lack of language translation, lack of health insurance, and lack of culturally competent health professionals, which only causes AANHPI women to distrust medical care, including for sexual and reproductive health care. "They have an extremely low rate of pap exams, resulting in a disproportionately high incidence of cervical cancer. Vietnamese have the highest rate of all ethnic groups, which is almost five times higher than white women" (Nakae, 2007, p. 17). ACRJ also connects U.S. agribusiness use of the pesticide DDT (a synthetic organic compound used as an insecticide) in Hawai'i to the native Hawai'ian women having "one of the highest breast cancer rates in the world" (ACRJ, 2005, p. 4). The idea that Asian women are more petite physically and can do more detailed work such as sewing or assembling small electronic components (known as the "nimble fingers theory") or that they have skill in agricultural work based on their livelihoods prior to migrating to the U.S., may also add stress to their bodies or expose them to certain chemicals, resulting in physical disabilities including carpal tunnel syndrome, tendinitis, arthritis, or cancers (Burgel et al., 2004; Enloe, 2014). Living with disabilities is yet another risk amplified because of economic and racial disparities.

Reproductive justice is both collective in seeking justice for the community in the face of social assumptions and institutional barriers to adequate reproductive access and care, and individual in terms of enjoying autonomy over one's own body – including decisions about whether to pursue health care and treatments that are accessible. A significant aspect of reproductive and sexual health care, moreover, is being able to communicate about genetic and environmental conditions that may affect one's sexual and reproductive health, as well as overall health in general. For example, exposure to radiation because of nuclear testing in the Pacific Ocean or to pesticides due to working in or proximity to agricultural labor is relevant to the sexual and reproductive health of Pacific Islanders and Asian immigrants, particularly women and children but also to anyone wanting to have children. Open discussion about genetic physical and mental health disorders is just as important when that information is available. Knowing whether one's biological parent or close relatives have had histories of breast, cervical, ovarian, or uterine cancer is likewise important for cis persons to know and to share with their health care providers. Knowing what resources are accessible in the community and to the community (e.g., via language translation) in order to better be able to process this knowledge is also essential. Being better informed as a community member and an individual is part of being able to make better decisions about one's health care. Being able to discuss sexual health also encourages women to be aware of their sexual partners' health history and make informed decisions about their sexual activities.

Having autonomy over one's own body moreover is relevant for AANHPI women making decisions about having children, sex or gender-affirming surgery. AANHPI community members of course hold diverse opinions about the circumstances under which they support abortion rights, sexual activity, or surgery to affirm one's gender identity. Yet it is important to remember that acts of anti-Asian violence and violence targeting AANHPI women are deeply connected to the ways groups of people have been and continue to be differentiated from each other – by presumed differences of race, sexuality, mental and physical abilities, gender expression, socioeconomic status, religious freedom, nationality, and other classifications. This differentiation often affects those who are perceived to not belong: they may suffer and have less access to resources, choices, and the ability to make choices for themselves. And those who have the power to label those different from themselves as less valuable only accumulate greater power and resources. This is why affirming bodily autonomy means ensuring that conditions in which individuals can make such decisions for themselves without coercion are absolutely about reproductive justice.

Why Is This Book Needed?

> Well, I'm sure it's probably different with them, but for me because I've kind of been more Americanized, I am more free – I talk with them freely. But when I go with my mom, and she has to say stuff, I'm the one who does the interpretation between the doctors and my parents. And so, they're very hush hush and they're very hesitant to share information. ... It's hard. It's hard because it's always been taboo. It's something you don't talk about. And so for them even when it comes to health, and it's something that has to be shared, they are really still very resistant about sharing.
>
> *-Bev, Focus group participant*

Historical and social factors inform how AANHPI women understand themselves, and this perception of who they are as women also affects their sexual and reproductive health. In addition to the specific histories of Asian and Pacific Islander nations in relation to the United States, relevant details include generational differences and levels of acculturation, language barriers to health care and resources, and age – or where one is in the life cycle. Much of the literature about Asian American women's sexuality solely use female college students for their studies (Sindhu, 2021). As is the case for studies about women's sexuality in general, sexual health and activity for older AANHPI women are much less studied. This may reflect societal assumptions that women's sexual activity is closely associated with sexual reproductivity and that sexual activity declines with menopause.

As a majority of AANHPI women are foreign-born, one of the key explanations about AANHPI women's sexual activity is level of acculturation to a new country; the more acculturated they are to the U.S. culture, the more a woman is assumed to be sexually active (Brotto et al., 2005). Acculturation also relates to an individual's immigrant generation. A first-generation immigrant according to the U.S. Census Bureau is a person who foreign-born. The second generation refers to children of immigrant parents who are born in the United States. The 1.5 generation refers to those who migrate to a new country during their early teens. While the acculturation explanation – how AANHPI women's health changes with more time spent in the United States – can be informative, relying solely on culture as an explanation overlooks the importance of larger social contexts including structural barriers (Viruell-Fuentes et al., 2012; Viruell-Fuentes & Schulz, 2009).

Larger social contexts matter, and the context of community in which AANHPI women live also relates to sexual and reproductive health. AANHPI women who accompanied their military husbands to the United States, for example, may have experienced isolation from a familiar culture if they resided on military bases or if they married non-Asian men. Studies of AANHPI war brides during the 1950s through 1970s reveal that many women felt scrutinized and treated like outsiders by the military community and the husbands' families. Although community often is assumed to be a positive factor and provide social support, communities may at times inhibit one's freedom to explore one's sexuality. Patriarchal cultures that assign shame to sexually active unmarried women will often result in community surveillance (Hunjan & Towson, 2007). Non-heterosexual AANHPI women may not feel that they can openly reveal their intimate relationships due to fears of community rejection and even violence (Choudhury, 2007). This has significance when it comes to medical care because AANHPI women who may not be comfortable communicating in English often rely upon family or community members during their medical appointments. Children most often translate for their parents, but even relying on a community member for translation may prevent women from asking about health concerns.

In some communities, however, same-sex relationships and sexual activity outside of marriage are not perceived so negatively. Native Hawaiians for example deeply value extended networks of extended families and friends. Large multi-generational households are not simply a reflection of socioeconomic status but reflect close familial relationships and cultural preferences (Soon et al., 2015). While unintended pregnancy might bring shame and disgrace to some Asian American communities (Holliday et al., 2017), the emphasis on family and children for Native Hawaiians may "lessen the burden of an unplanned pregnancy (Soon et al., 2015, p. 166)", because children are "a blessing upon the entire o'hana (Soon et al., 2015, p. 167)". This cannot be easily generalized however, because additional factors including religious affiliation can also make a difference (Hasnain et al., 2020).

One segment among AANHPI women who must be included when it comes to issues of sexual and reproductive health are those living with disabilities. Research shows that Asian Americans are underrepresented in research about disabilities. Hasnain et al. (2020) note, "Asian Americans – on individual, family, and group levels are overlooked and ignored; their diversity is oversimplified, and they are treated as a homogeneous entity in research, especially in studies focused on disabilities." People with physical disabilities often are assumed to lack sexuality, just as those who identify as asexual are assumed to "have something wrong with them." Sexual activity and biological reproduction historically have assumed the domain of able-bodied persons (Kim et al., 2021). Open dialogue about sexual and reproductive health requires awareness that people with disabilities often have their sexuality denied, and access to sexual activity and reproductive rights diminished. This lack of access is also part of AANHPI history.

Because of the impossibility of generalizing across diverse AANHPI cultures or even within ethnic groups, the role of community members who are knowledgeable about specific ethnic communities in specific locations is critical for health care outreach and/or research. Health researchers and health education programs have noted the importance of recruiting respected community members to serve as "cultural brokers" in reaching racial and ethnic minority and/or low-income groups. "Unlike physicians and nurses, community navigators do not provide healthcare services directly; they offer culturally tailored educational support to patients, aid communication between patients and physicians, and guide patients in overcoming barriers to obtaining appropriate healthcare" (Shommu et al., 2016, p. 2). One review of efforts to increase cancer screenings, found community health navigators (CHNs) to be effective for encouraging screening participation among various racial minority and disadvantaged communities, largely due to their familiarity with and acceptance within their local groups" (Hou & Roberson, 2015, p. 173). In the case of these screenings, the CHNs were trained specifically about the particular health intervention either in a one-day session or several-day sessions to make the materials more relevant and accessible to communities. For clinic settings, patients who interacted with CHNs were more likely to complete the screening (Hou & Roberson, 2015).

Most of the literature about community navigators addressed health care interventions relating to diabetes, heart disease, or cancer, and very few focused on Asian American communities. In a systemic review of research investigating the effectiveness of community navigator intervention among immigrant populations, specifically for chronic disease management; Shommu and colleagues (2016) found that only four out of 103 research focused on Asian American communities. Culturally tailored interventions for Chinese American women to encourage mammography screening for breast cancer (which is lower than other Asian groups) included educators who shared the same background. Studies found that this outreach helped address fears about the process and limited English ability (Zhang et al., 2020). None addressed reproductive health. However, women's clinics related to sexual and reproductive health located within underserved, predominantly racial minority, and lower-income neighborhoods may already rely on trusted community members in their outreach but may not contribute to studies and research that are grant- or research-based.

The Reproductive Justice model already assumes that community members possess the expertise to work with and advocate for their communities. As Toni Bond of African American Women Evolving states, "Reproductive justice clarifies the ways that women's decisions are shaped by unequal access to power and resources, by the environment, by economics, by culture" (Bond, 2007, p. 15). The growing population and diversity of AANHPI communities in the United States will require understanding about the inequalities that result in differential access to the resources needed to reduce and eliminate racial inequities in sexual and reproductive health.

Although not a major focus, this book also illustrates transdisciplinary collaboration with community partnership. The first chapter draws from media studies and literature; the second chapter uses demographic methods; the third chapter uses storytelling to talk about sexual and reproductive health of AANHPI women.

The Arizona Asian American and Pacific Islander Women's Health Project

> I will say as I learned more about sexual health as an adult, I was rather annoyed that I didn't know more about it younger. Especially when I started doing online courses and learning and I learned, Oh! Sex could have been so much better! I was robbed! [laughter all around] Years!
>
> -*Roseanne, Focus group participant*

To address the lack of inclusion of AANHPI women's sexual and reproductive health in the current research, the authors began the Arizona Asian American and Pacific Islander Women's Health Project to document AANHPI women's experiences with respect to health, particularly sexual and reproductive health. With a grant from the Arizona State University Institute for Humanities Research that brings researchers together from different disciplinary backgrounds, we designed a study that combined research from the humanities and the social sciences. Our project not only sought to look at the disaggregation of AANHPI data on women's health, but also review the ways in which historical context and literature frame the sexual and reproductive health of AANHPI women. In addition, we wanted to utilize a methodology that included storytelling, because memories of how we learn about sex and reproduction may shape the choices made about health. The grant from the Institute for Humanities Research allowed us to conduct focus groups and collect surveys, and hold a public event to present some of the themes from our work to the community members.

Our research drew heavily on elements of community-based research, where we worked through community events and with community leaders to discuss the reasons for the project and to recruit for our focus group participants. Because health care providers often rely on medical research studies for their knowledge, we seek to amplify these underrepresented experiences that are vastly important for understanding how knowledge about sexual and reproductive health is generated in cross-cultural and intergenerational ways.

We limited our data collection to Maricopa County and, in order to counter the heavy emphasis in the literature on college-age AANHPI women, we intentionally focused on participants who were 25 years of age or older. We also sought AANHPI women participants who represented different ethnic backgrounds, immigration experiences and generations. Although the AANHPI population in Arizona is the fastest growing ethnic minority population in the state, it comprises just 6% of the total population and is most heavily concentrated in Maricopa County (APIA Vote, 2022). The largest AA groups are Filipino, Asian Indian, and Chinese (excluding Taiwanese) and nearly 18% of the AA population in Arizona is foreign-born (MPI, 2021). In addition to Native Hawaiians, the largest PI groups are CHamoru and Sāmoan. Focus group participants included nearly all these groups, as well as individuals of Japanese, Korean, and Vietnamese backgrounds. Even with our attempt to ensure a wide range of AANHPI community members, we were limited in our ability to provide translation and interpretation, so all of our participants used English to participate in the focus group discussions, even if English was not their preferred language. A community elder provided some help with interpretation and translation of colloquialisms and phrases for some participants during one focus group discussion.

For the focus groups, we recruited participants through community events and spreading the word through our networks via email lists and social media. Most of our initial outreach was done via AANHPI festivals. We set up a booth and did outreach at the local "Matsuri: Celebration of Japan" festival, a decades-old tradition held in downtown Phoenix. We also recruited participants at the Arizona Aloha Festival, a large event highlighting Pacific Islander culture in Arizona. Our outreach was intended both to have general conversations about health and to ask attendees if they would be interested in participating in our project. In order to initiate conversations, we used a big board with the question, "What does HEALTH mean to you?" in the middle of the board. We used colorful sticky notes to draw festival attendees to our booth and began a conversation about health, and invited them to write a sentence or phrase to express what health meant to them. Over the course of four days of festivals, hundreds of people of all ages stopped by to add a phrase and talk with us about our project. We received one-word responses such as "Happy" and "Life" and phrases such as "Everything! Living longer, family & friends, smiling" and "Being happy. Emotionally, mentally."

After discussing our project, we provided flyers and a sign-up sheet for more information and recruited over a dozen participants through these means. In order to personalize our ask, we included our photos on the flyer and the physical address of where focus groups would be held, at the site of a community health organization. We also sent out the request through our networks, and one community leader independently recruited almost 10 Pacific Islander participants through her connections. Overall, we held four focus groups with participation ranging from three to 10 women in each group, with a total of 24 participants. Each focus group discussion lasted one hour followed by a short, written survey. See Appendix A for the focus group script and survey questions.

The authors knew or worked with some of the participants in other capacities in the community, which may have allowed for a level of comfort in some of the focus groups. The community leader who recruited participants to take part accompanied them to three of the four focus groups (acting as a participant herself in one of the groups), which may have led to additional levels of trust in the process. We were surprised that although many of the stories featured elements of shame and punishment, they were told with humor – the women in our focus groups echoed each other's experiences, layering their telling, encouraging and supporting each other, and laughing at the ways in which they were taught about sex and their bodies. The openness with which they shared the stories was somewhat unexpected for us, given that these were topics rarely discussed by their families. Many women wanted to stay together beyond the focus group to continue the conversation and expressed gratitude to have space to talk about topics they said they do not often openly talk about.

We note that the community-based recruitment model (including through churches and established community organizations) may have had unexpected consequences, including the lack of participation of any individuals who identified as non-heterosexual or transgender. A dominant observation among Asian American scholars of queer studies is the ways in which Asian American community organizations often organize with a focus on ethnic identity; the lack of attention to sexual or gender diversity often results in assumptions of heterosexuality (Alvarez et al., 2020; Kumashiro, 2004; Naber, 2006). In communities like Arizona with relatively few AANHPI organizations, queer and transgender AANHPIs may identify more with queer and transgender organizations. Generational differences also may have been a factor. Our intent to recruit participants older than 25 with ethnic diversity may have contributed to less sexual and gender diversity, or less willingness to claim non-heterosexuality among other community members. Some of the findings from our research are discussed throughout the book, particularly in Chapters 2 and 3. The public event we hosted for AANHPI community members to learn about our findings utilized humor as a key component. For that we worked with performance artist Kristina Wong to creatively approach ways that our research findings and individual experiences could be integrated. We discuss this approach in the final chapter.

We hope this book will generate further conversations among AANHPI women about sexual and reproductive health and expand how both researchers and health providers approach serving these populations. We were encouraged by the responses and support we received from the women who spoke with us. As one of the focus group participants said, "I think just to come here to hear what you guys [are] sharing, it really makes me excited. It's the first time for me to attend this kind of meeting with *all* women."

Notes

1 Because reproductive health is an integral part of women's sexual health, as discussed later in this chapter, we use the terms "sexual and reproductive health" and "sexual health" interchangeably throughout the manuscript.

2 Asian Americans refers to those with Asian heritage who either immigrated to or were born in the United States. Native Hawaiian acknowledges those who are descended from persons indigenous to Hawai`i prior to colonization and U.S. statehood. Pacific Islanders also refers to those descended from persons indigenous to the Pacific Islands. Indigenous Pacific Islanders Please see https://www.govinfo.gov/content/pkg/FR-1997-10-30/pdf/97-28653.pdf, particularly p. 58785-58787 for the U.S. government's decision to create two categories,

"Asian" and "Native Hawaiian or Other Pacific Islander". The shift from Asian Americans and Pacific Islanders (AANHPI) occurred after the 2000 US Census, although the umbrella AANHPI category is still prevalently used in practice.

3 AANHPI rates of mental illness and distress are higher than the general population and AANPHIs demonstrate lower rates of utilizing mental health care resources (SAMHSA, 2022). The Asian American Psychological Association also annually updates fact sheets about mental health concerns for Asian Americans.

4 We have used pseudonyms throughout the book and have chosen not to provide detailed descriptions of the individuals quoted due to the small network of AANHPI in Maricopa County who might be able to attribute quotes to specific individuals.

References

Abrams, A. (2019). 'We are grabbing our own microphones': How advocates of reproductive justice stepped into the spotlight. *Time*. Retrieved from https://time.com/5735432/reproductive-justice-groups/

Alvarez, A. R., Kanuha, V. K., Anderson, M. K., Kapua, C., & Bifulco, K. (2020). "We Were Queens." Listening to Kānaka Maoli Perspectives on Historical and On-Going Losses in Hawai'i. *Genealogy*, *4*(4), 116. 10.3390/genealogy4040116

Asian Communities for Reproductive Justice (ACRJ), (2005). *A new vision for advancing our movement for reproductive health, reproductive rights and reproductive justice*. Retrieved from https://forwardtogether.org/wp-content/uploads/2017/12/ACRJ-A-New-Vision.pdf

Asian and Pacific Islander American Vote (APIAVote), (2022). *APIA voter demographics by state: Arizona*. Retrieved from https://apiavote.org/wp-content/uploads/Arizona.pdf

Bond, T. M. (2007). Reproductive justice and women of color. *SisterSong Women of Color Reproductive Health Collective. The Reproductive Justice Briefing Book: A Primer on Reproductive Justice and Social Change.* Retrieved from https://www.law.berkeley.edu/php-programs/courses/fileDL.php?fID=4051.

Braveman, P., & Gottlieb, L. (2014). The social determinants of health: It's time to consider the causes of the causes. *Public Health Reports*, *129*(1_suppl2), 19–31. 10.1177/00333549141291S206

Brotto, L. A., Chik, H. M., Ryder, A. G., Gorzalka, B. B., & Seal, B. N. (2005). Acculturation and sexual function in Asian women. *Archives of sexual Behavior*, *34*, 613–626. 10.1007/s10508-005-7909-6

Burgel, B. J., Lashuay, N., Israel, L., & Harrison, R. (2004). Garment workers in California: health outcomes of the Asian Immigrant Women Workers Clinic. *AAOHN Journal*, *52*(11), 465–475. 10.1177/216507990405201106

Center for Population Health. (2020). What is Population Health? https://www.cdc.gov/pophealthtraining/whatis.html

Chou, R. S. (2012). *Asian American sexual politics: the construction of race, gender, and sexuality*. Rowman & Littlefield.

Choudhury, P. P. (2007). *The Violence That Dares Not Speak Its Name: Invisibility in the lives of lesbian and bisexual South Asian American women. In S.D. Dasgupta (Ed.), Body Evidence: intimate violence against South Asian women in America* (pp. 126-138). Rutgers University Press.

Edwards, W. M., & Coleman, E. (2004). Defining sexual health: A descriptive overview. *Archives of Sexual Behavior*, *33*, 189–195. 10.1023/B:ASEB.0000026619.95734.d5

Enloe, C. (2014). *Bananas, beaches and bases: Making feminist sense of international politics*. Berkeley CA: University of California Press.
Hasnain, R., Fujiura, G. T., Capua, J. E., Bui, T. T. T., & Khan, S. (2020). Disaggregating the Asian "other": Heterogeneity and methodological issues in research on Asian Americans with disabilities. *Societies*, *10*(3), 58. 10.3390/soc 10030058
"health." Merriam-Webster.com. (2023). https://www.merriam-webster.com/dictionary/health#citations
Hillman, J. (2011). A call for an integrated biopsychosocial model to address fundamental disconnects in an emergent field: An introduction to the special issue on "Sexuality and Aging". *Ageing International*, *36*, 303–312. 10.1007/s12126-011-9122-3
Holliday, C. N., McCauley, H. L., Silverman, J. G., Ricci, E., Decker, M. R., Tancredi, D. J., ... & Miller, E. (2017). Racial/ethnic differences in women's experiences of reproductive coercion, intimate partner violence, and unintended pregnancy. *Journal of Women's Health*, *26*(8), 828–835. 10.1089/jwh.2016.5996
Hou, S.L., & Roberson, K. (2015). A systematic review on US-based community health navigator (CHN) interventions for cancer screening promotion—comparing community-versus clinic-based navigator models. *Journal of Cancer Education*, *30*, 173–186. 10.1007/s13187-014-0723-x
Hunjan, S., & Towson, S. (2007). "Virginity is Everything": Sexuality in the Context of Intimate Partner Violence in the South Asian Community. In S. D. Dasgupta (Ed.), *Body evidence* pp. *53-67*.
Kim, J. B., Kupetz, J., Lie, C. Y., & Cynthia, W. (2021). *Sex, identity, aesthetics: The work of Tobin Siebers and disability studies*. University of Michigan Press.
Kindig, D., & Stoddart, G. (2003). What is population health? *American Journal of Public Health*, *93*(3), 380–383. 10.2105/AJPH.93.3.380
Kochiyama, Y., Lee, M., Kochiyama-Sardinha, A., & Kochiyama-Holman, A. (2004). *Passing it on: A memoir*. University of California Los Angeles Asian American Studies Center Press.
Kumashiro, K. K. (2004). *Restoried selves: Autobiographies of queer Asian-Pacific-American activists*. Psychology Press.
Lantz, P. M., Lichtenstein, R. L., & Pollack, H. A. (2007). Health policy approaches to population health: The limits of medicalization. *Health Affairs*, *26*(5), 1253–1257. 10.1377/hlthaff.26.5.1253
Lindau, S. T., Laumann, E. O., Levinson, W., & Waite, L. J. (2003). Synthesis of scientific disciplines in pursuit of health: The interactive biopsychosocial model. *Perspectives in biology and medicine*, *46*(3 Suppl), S74–S84. 10.1353/pbm.2003.0055
Link, B. G., & Phelan, J. (1995). Social conditions as fundamental causes of disease. *Journal of Health and Social Behavior*, 80–94. 10.2307/2626958
Mendenhall, E. (2016). *Syndemic Suffering: Social distress, depression, and diabetes among Mexican immigrant women* (Vol. 4). Routledge.
Migration Policy Institute. (2021). *State immigration data profiles: Arizona*. Retrieved from https://www.migrationpolicy.org/data/state-profiles/state/demographics/AZ
Naber, N. (2006). Arab American femininities: Beyond Arab virgin/American (ized) whore. *Feminist studies*, *32*(1), 87–111. 10.2307/20459071
Nakae, M. (2007). Reproductive justice issues for Asian and Pacific Islander women. In *Reproductive Justice Briefing Book: A Primer on Reproductive Justice and Social Change*.
Phelan, J. C., Link, B. G., & Tehranifar, P. (2010). Social conditions as fundamental causes of health inequalities: Theory, evidence, and policy

implications. *Journal of health and social behavior*, *51*(1_suppl), S28–S40. 10.1177/0022146510383498

Robinson, B. B., Bockting, W. O., Simon Rosser, B., Miner, M., & Coleman, E. (2002). The sexual health model: Application of a sexological approach to HIV prevention. *Health education research*, *17*(1), 43–57. 10.1093/her/17.1.43

Ross, L. J. (2007). *The Reproductive Justice Briefing Book: A Primer on Reproductive Justice and Social Change. Sistersong Women of Color Reproductive Health Collective*. Retrieved from https://www.law.berkeley.edu/php-programs/courses/fileDL.php?fID=4051.

Ross, L. J., Gutiérrez, E., Gerber, M., & Silliman, J. (2016). *Undivided rights: Women of color organizing for reproductive justice*. Haymarket Books.

SAMHSA. (2022). *Key substance use and mental health indicators in the United States: Results from the 2021 National Survey on Drug Use and Health*. Retrieved from https://www.samhsa.gov/data/report/2021-nsduh-annual-national-report

Sartorius, N. (2006). The meanings of health and its promotion. *Croatian Medical Journal*, *47*(4), 662.

Schalk, S., & Kim, J. B. (2020). Integrating race, transforming feminist disability studies. *Signs: Journal of Women in Culture and Society*, *46*(1), 31–55. 10.1086/718866

Shommu, N. S., Ahmed, S., Rumana, N., Barron, G. R., McBrien, K. A., & Turin, T. C. (2016). What is the scope of improving immigrant and ethnic minority healthcare using community navigators: A systematic scoping review. *International journal for equity in health*, *15*(1), 1–12. 10.1186/s12939-016-0298-8

Sindhu, P. (2021). Sexual health in the Asian-American population of the United States. *PCOM Capstone Projects. 38.* https://digitalcommons.pcom.edu/capstone_projects/38

Soon, R., Elia, J., Beckwith, N., Kaneshiro, B., & Dye, T. (2015). Unintended pregnancy in the Native Hawaiian community: Key informants' perspectives. *Perspectives on sexual and reproductive health*, *47*(4), 163–170. 10.1363/47e5615

Viruell-Fuentes, E. A., Miranda, P. Y., & Abdulrahim, S. (2012). More than culture: structural racism, intersectionality theory, and immigrant health. *Social science & medicine*, *75*(12), 2099–2106. 10.1016/j.socscimed.2011.12.037

Viruell-Fuentes, E. A., & Schulz, A. J. (2009). Toward a dynamic conceptualization of social ties and context: Implications for understanding immigrant and Latino health. *American journal of public health*, *99*(12), 2167–2175. https://ajph.aphapublications.org/doi/abs/10.2105/AJPH.2008.158956

Wang Kong, C., Green, J., Hamity, C., & Jackson, A. (2022). Health disparity measurement among Asian American, Native Hawaiian, and Pacific Islander populations across the United States. *Health Equity*, *6*(1), 533–539. 10.1089/heq.2022.0051

World Health Organization, (2002). Constitution of the World Health Organization. 1946. *Bulletin of the World Health Organization*, *80*(12), 983.

World Health Organization, (2006). *Defining sexual health: Report of a technical consultation on sexual health, 28-31 January 2002*, Geneva: World Health Organization.

Yamada, M. (1979). Invisibility is an unnatural disaster: Reflections of an Asian American Woman. *Bridge, An Asian American Perspective*, *7*(1), 11–13.

Zhang, X., Li, P., Guo, P., Wang, J., Liu, N., Yang, S., … & Zhang, W. (2020). Culturally tailored intervention to promote mammography screening practice among Chinese American women: a systematic review. *Journal of Cancer Education*, *35*, 1052–1060. 10.1007/s13187-020-01730-4

1 Historic and Gendered Representations: Asian Americans and Pacific Islanders, Real and Imagined

Who Are Asian Americans and Pacific Islanders?

> I only found out decades later when my Aunt Helen, leaning forward and dropping her voice, confided in me, "You know she talked to her first doctor."
>
> "What?" I leaned forward too.
>
> "She told the doctor she felt something in her breast."
>
> "She did?"
>
> "Yes. And he laughed it off. Said, 'You women are all alike.' That was a few years before she was diagnosed."
>
> My mother died three years from breast cancer after she finally was diagnosed. Could she have survived had the doctor not shrugged off her concerns? Could she have survived had she felt empowered to challenge the doctor's authority?
>
> And who was the "you" in "you women" – was it all women? Was it all Asian American women?
>
> We women are not all alike. And acknowledging this maybe a matter of life or death.
>
> *-Amy, third-generation Chinese American daughter*
>
> But, coming here to America, 'cause I grew up in Hawai'i … . that transition was really really hard for us. And trying to understand.
>
> *-Fran, Focus group participant*

Asian Americans and Pacific Islanders are a diverse population. Asian Americans include citizens and residents of varying legal status in the United States who identify as having Asian descent (J. Lee & Ramakrishnan, 2020). The U.S. Census defines this as persons having origins in East Asia, Southeast Asia, the Indian Subcontinent, or parts of West Asia. The majority (94%) of Asian Americans originate from or claim ancestry from 19 Asian countries, which themselves are comprised of multiple language, ethnic, and religious groups (J. Lee & Ramakrishnan, 2020). Some Asian Americans are themselves or descendants of voluntary

DOI: 10.4324/9781003449867-2

migrants to the United States, beginning from the mid-19th century, while other groups are refugees from political conflicts. In contrast, Pacific Islanders have been incorporated into the United States as a result of U.S. imperialism and colonization throughout the Pacific. Pacific Islanders are the descendants of the original inhabitants of the Pacific regions including Polynesia (e.g., Hawai'i, Sāmoa, and Tonga), Melanesia (e.g., Fiji and Vanuatu), and Micronesia (e.g., Guåhan, Marshall Islands, and Chuuk) (Kaholokula et al., 2019).

Asian Americans are also the fastest growing population in the United States since 2000; Native Hawaiian and Pacific Islanders are the second fastest growing population. In 2019, Americans of Asian descent alone constituted 5.9%, and Native Hawaiian and Other Pacific Islanders alone constituted 0.2% of the United States population. The majority of Asian Americans in the United States are foreign-born as about two out of three Asian Americans are immigrants. In 2019, the foreign-born Asian Americans and Pacific Islanders were nearly 60% of the total AANHPI population (U.S. Census Bureau, 2019).

The prominence of the U.S. military in the Pacific resulted in migration in the United States due to economic and intimate relations (Loyd et al., 2016). However, Pacific Islanders have varying relationships with the United States. Hawai`i is the only Pacific Island that is a state, and hence, Kānaka Maoli (as Native Hawaiians refer to themselves) and other Pacific Islanders born in Hawai'i are considered U.S. citizens by the United States. Other Pacific Islanders may enter the United States from unincorporated territories (i.e., American Sāmoa, Guåhan – referred to by the U.S. as Guam, Mariana Islands) or from nations who are part of the 1985 Compact of Free Association (COFA) that granted former U.S. territories their own sovereign status (i.e., Federated States of Micronesia, Republic of the Marshall Islands, and Republic of Palau). Pacific Islanders not from Hawai`i have varying levels of citizenship or status with the United States as a result: individuals born in Guåhan and the Northern Mariana Islands are U.S. citizens but do not have the right to vote in federal elections. Those born in American Samoa are U.S. nationals, not citizens; like citizens of U.S. territories, they cannot vote in federal elections. Individuals with citizenship in the COFA nations may travel to the United States as nonimmigrants without visas.

Even with these unique immigration histories, cultures, modes of entry, and policy contexts; AANHPIs began organizing in the 1960s and 1970s as a panethnic group with shared political interests (Espiritu, 1993; Omi & Winant, 1994). Common experiences of being treated differently due to being seen as foreign and not American contributed to a sense of collective interests (Espiritu, 1993; Zia, 2000). However, this panethnic political identity also contributes to an ongoing assumption among many Americans that "Asian Pacific American" is a monolithic racial category that groups Asian ethnic groups together; this in turn legitimizes the misconception of homogeneity among Asian Pacific Americans (Hollinger, 2006). Pacific Islanders increasingly have resisted this categorization because their distinct colonial histories and sovereign status so often have been and continue to be overlooked by Asian Americans. Several Pacific Islander communities have sought for decades to distinguish their relationship with the United States as involuntary; they only achieved a distinct group status in 1997 with the revision of racial and ethnic categories by the U.S. Office of Management and Business (OMB). The racial category, "Native Hawaiian and Other Pacific Islander" was first included in the 2000 decennial Census (Sasa & Yellow Horse, 2022).

An intersectional analysis of AANHPI diversity reveals further distinctions based on educational attainment, income, and wealth. The term intersectionality was first introduced by Black feminist legal scholar Kimberlé Crenshaw in the 1980s to address the inability of the U.S. legal system to address how Black women face both sexist and racist discrimination at the same time (Crenshaw, 2021). The law only allowed for either race or gender discrimination. The use of intersectionality has since broadened considerably to convey that women's experiences are influenced not only by their gender but also by other factors, including biological sex, sexual orientation, race and ethnicity, class status, and other factors like religion, region, or citizenship status. While one's social location is therefore always a combination of factors, intersectionality clearly reveals how inequalities have emerged from U.S. institutions like the law. For example, U.S. citizenship historically included some and excluded others based on these social factors. The first naturalization law in 1790 only allowed foreign-born persons who were White, male, and free to become U.S. citizens. This law excluded foreign-born White females, non-White males, and non-White females from becoming U.S. citizens. Exclusion from citizenship meant a lack of direct protection under U.S. law; a White woman had no individual vote in elections because her White husband or father was assumed to represent her interests. Thus, anyone who lacked the full rights of citizenship did not enjoy the power to act in their own interests, and was not fully recognized as belonging in U.S. society.

Even now that naturalized citizenship has been extended equally to all who qualify regardless of gender or race, not all persons have equal access to citizenship nor enjoy citizenship equally. Some people born elsewhere may lack equal access to securing U.S. citizenship because they may not have the money to pay for legal representation, which often hastens the process. This lack of equal access reflects a lack of equity. Finally, due to racism, sexism, homophobia, ableism, classism, and other forms of discrimination enacted in society, even persons who have birthright or naturalized citizenship may not feel fully welcomed in society, meaning that they experience what is called secondary citizenship. The vast diversity among Asian Americans and Pacific Islanders reflects differential access, opportunities, and inclusion in the national community, as can be seen in the history of Asian and Pacific Islanders in the United States.

From 1875 to 1965, immigration from Asia and the Pacific Islands was restricted due to race-based quotas that favored Northern European nations. After the 1965 Immigration and Naturalization Act removed these national limits, Asian migration to the United States rapidly increased with "the fastest population growth rate of any racial or ethnic group from 1990 to 2019" (Budiman & Ruiz, 2021). This 1965 legislation instituted categories based on skilled and unskilled labor, family reunification, and refugee status (Hing, 1993). As a result, some Asian Americans entering the United States have entered under H1B visas for in-demand, highly skilled labor or with EB-5 visas (created in 1990) for entrepreneurs who invest at least one million dollars in a startup business that will hire at least ten employees (Zhou & Lee, 2017). Those immigrants considered to be "less skilled" and less wealthy have entered under family reunification categories or refugee status; without legal counsel and guidance, some may wait for up to 20 years to achieve permanent residency.

Today, differences among AANHPIs continue to shape their relationships with the United States. Not all AANHPIs desire U.S. citizenship. Some Asians came to the United States because they were fleeing political persecution and identify as refugees, not voluntary migrants. Most Asian arrivals to the United States have been motivated because of economic, religious, and/or political pressures within their communities of origin. Second-generation Asian Americans born in the United States who have birthright U.S. citizenship may have a very different perspective than the immigrant first generation.

Nonetheless, Asian immigrants' ability to be in the United States (and U.S. territories in the Pacific or elsewhere) is a result of U.S. imperialism and the subsequent taking by force of lands and resources from Indigenous populations who initially inhabited those places. Asian Americans share with Kānaka Maoli and Pacific Islanders a common experience of lacking full social inclusion because of their racialized identities. But they are also differentiated by the political distinction and material dispossession experienced by Kānaka Maoli and Pacific Islanders. Some Kānaka Maoli for example have organized politically around the return of Hawaiian sovereignty and separation from the United States, while others do not see the restoration of a sovereign Hawaiian nation as economically or politically viable (Goodyear-Kaopua et al., 2014; Pacheco, 2010). Pacific Islanders likewise may differ in their responses to the United States' military and economic dominance over their nations that has resulted from U.S. colonization (Niumeitolu, 2015; Salinas, 2020).

AANHPI Women

In 2019, the estimated population of Asian American women was 10,197,257, with the majority of women 25–44 years old (2,687,046 making up 26.3% of AA women) or 45 years old and older (2,878,102 making up 28.2% of AA women) (U.S. Census Bureau, 2019). Fewer than 2 million Asian American females are 18 years old and younger (less than 20% of AA women). In contrast, Pacific Islander females 45 years old or older are estimated at 86,861 persons, while those 25–44 years old are 103,691 and those under 18 years old are nearly 100,000 (U.S. Census Bureau, 2019). Among Asian American LGBT adults, half are women in contrast to 56% of Native Hawaiian Pacific Islander LGBT adults (Choi, 2021).

These AANHPI demographic characteristics show the importance of understanding AANHPI women's sexual and reproductive health across the life span and for all age groups; language fluency likely will continue to be a factor in health outreach and education given the large number of foreign-born AANHPI women. Yet, most of the research on AANHPI women's sexual and reproductive health focuses on college-aged women, the majority of whom are fluent in English and selected based on educational attainment (meaning, research also excludes "college-aged" (e.g., emerging adults from ages 18 to 25) women who are not in higher education). Limited knowledge, combined with cultural reticence to speak about sexual health and popular stereotypes about AANHPI female sexuality, pose challenges for promoting sexual and reproductive health among AANHPI women.

AANHPI Women as Imagined by the United States and U.S. Society

> For me, because I kind of grew up in both worlds, I learned … to take the good and leave the bad. … And that goes for sex education, it goes with everything really – diet, everything single thing. … we have to learn to be able to adapt better with this lifestyle … not to totally leave behind our island ways and totally take up American ways. But to take the good of both.
>
> *-Fran, Focus group participant*

As noted earlier, AANHPI women and men experience racism and colonization differently because of specific cultural expectations in both their homelands and the United States. Several feminist scholars over the past three decades have explored how Asian American as well as Kānaka Maoli and Pacific Islander women have been known and understood in American society (Desmond, 1997; Espiritu, 1997; Fojas, 2014; Imada,

2012; Konzett, 2017; Marchetti, 1994; Shimizu, 2007; Silva, 2004; Yamamoto, 1999). Kānaka Maoli and Pacific Islanders were colonized by European and then U.S. imperialisms that imposed foreign political power and cultural values upon their communities. Hawai'i was annexed in 1899 and became a U.S. state in 1959, but some Native Hawaiians continue to fight for the return of their sovereignty in the present. In contrast, most Asian Americans chose to migrate to the United States and are subject to immigration policies, even though those choices may have been due to economic and political pressures exerted by the U.S. and European powers upon their Asian homelands that "pushed" them to migrate.

Pacific Islanders were perceived as different and less civilized from the very moment of contact by European explorers. European exploration was based on identifying new sources of materials to enrich the political, economic, and military power of their homelands and expand their territorial claims globally. Beginning in the 15th century, Micronesia, Polynesia, and Melanesia were targeted for colonization and passed through claims by Spain, the Dutch, Great Britain, Germany, the United States, Japan and New Zealand, over the course of four centuries of war and conflict. Different cultural ideas about nudity and clothing immediately resulted in European explorers assuming that Pacific Islander cultures were more promiscuous because the women did not cover their breasts. Royal Navy commander James Cook's expeditions through the Pacific Islands often are credited with spreading this narrative of sexually available Pacific Islander women throughout the world (Imada, 2012). Although in Polynesian cultures women's ability to bear children elevated their status in the community, and several women were recognized as leaders, European colonization assumed a diminished role while viewing Pacific Islander women as highly sexualized objects of desire (Imada, 2012; McDougall, 2016; McGregor, 2003). This sexualization – perceiving women as sexual objects for sexual pleasure – continues today with the "hula girl" stereotype promoted by tourism, which constitutes a major industry for the Pacific Islands. Although the hula girl depicted is seen as a foreign, seductive woman, the practice of hula is a highly spiritual practice for Native Hawaiians that tells stories of creation, gods, and relations among all beings (McDougall, 2016). The strategic locations of the Pacific Islands and some Asian nations as bases for naval security in the Pacific Rim have also resulted in high rates of prostitution at port towns to service military personnel, which may provide more wages for some women than other wage work (Bailey & Farber, 1994; Moon, 1997).

Like the European explorers of the Pacific Islands, U.S. diplomats and missionaries to Asia in the 19th century looked to social relations between men and women to index their own civilization. Reports of the bound feet of Chinese women, the exotic geisha in Japan who entertained male customers, and other stories of different cultural practices resulted in Asians being perceived as inherently different and less civilized than Americans. Increased Asian immigration to the United States beginning in the mid-19th century inspired fears of vast numbers of Asians overtaking the United States or a "Yellow Peril" – the Western fear that Asians would invade their lands and disrupt Western values (Chan, 1991a). Whites assigned Asians as immoral as evidenced by their lack of Christian values, poor treatment of women (e.g., foot binding of women), and addiction to opium. In fact, the first immigration law to restrict any group on the basis of race was the 1875 Page Law. While overall the purpose of the law was to prohibit entry to contract labor from "China, Japan, or any other Oriental country," the first section of the law specifically affirmed Americans' assumptions that Asian female immigrants to the United States were being imported involuntarily as prostitutes (Chan, 1991a). The law authorized U.S. officials at any port in Asia to screen U.S.–bound female passengers (Chan, 1991a) to determine where they had "entered into a contract or agreement for a term of service … for lewd and immoral purposes" (Abrams, 2005; Chan, 1991b). If officials doubted their moral character, they could deny entry into the United States. The presence of Chinese bachelor societies and the lack of wives and families contributed to prejudicial assumptions that the Chinese did not value families. As the Anti-Chinese movement pundits in the western states argued throughout the 1870s and 1880s, this lack of family values allowed Chinese male labor to work for less wages. This in turn would drive European American working men out of jobs, force their wives and daughters into prostitution and servitude, and corrupt their sons with a lack of industry and an abundance of prostitutes (Leong, 2001). These federal laws preventing the immigration of Asian women – or what Miliann Kang describes as "reproductive exclusion" (Kang, 2020) – significantly slowed the emergence of U.S.-born Asian American communities.

Viewing Asians as inherently different also led to multiple competing stereotypes about Asian American women. Yen Le Espiritu has categorized feminine stereotypes of Asian American women as a sweet, innocent and submissive Lotus Blossom archetype (also known as the China Doll), or the aggressive and seductive Dragon Lady who manipulates men with her sexuality (Espiritu, 1997). The fragile female subject to dominant Asian patriarchs is not as prominent in popular depictions, except when in need of rescue, often but not always by non-Asian men or governments. The 2003 film *Crash*, known for revealing the humanity of a multicultural cast of morally complex characters except for the Asian American men trafficking Asian immigrant women in Chinatown, is one example. The rare example of a romance between an Asian American man and woman in the 1961 musical *Flower Drum*

Song involves Mei Li, an innocent young immigrant woman new to the United States, capturing the heart of Wang Ta, a culturally confused Asian American male who pines after a modern Americanized showgirl. Another example of a romance between an Asian American man and woman is from the recent 2018 film, *Crazy Rich Asians*. Asian American women and Pacific Islander women commonly have been hypersexualized in American popular culture. Numerous examples include but are not limited to early photographs of Chinese women labeled as Chinese prostitutes in San Francisco to a Japanese American woman accused of being the seductive Tokyo Rose during World War II, and to the aforementioned Hawaiian hula girls to depictions of sex workers in a series of films set in Vietnam.

These historical perceptions of Asian American and Pacific Islander women, developed from the earliest contact of European explorers with Asian and Pacific Islander cultures continue to inform the ways in which AANHPI women are portrayed in popular representations such as movies even into the present. In addition to the sexualized, gendered, and racialized stereotypes described above, AANHPI women rarely have been portrayed onscreen as complex characters. For example, a 2021 study examined the number of AANHPI characters as well as the prominence of the roles in the 100 most popular Hollywood films annually from 2007 to 2019 (Yuen et al., 2021). According to Yuen and colleagues, only 3.4% of the 1,300 top-grossing films in this 13-year period featured AANHPI leads or co-leads. Among them, even fewer – only six of the AANHPI lead roles equating less than 1/10th of a percent – were AANHPI women. The absence of AANHPI women from Hollywood films as developed characters is connected to the ways that AANHPI women have been excluded as members of American society. One-third of the six AANHPI roles (only two roles) were animated young female characters. The only NHPI lead among the six roles was the protagonist of the Disney animated film, *Moana*, voiced by Auli'i Carvalho, who since that role has identified as a member of the LGBTQ+ community. Chloe Bennet voiced the leading role of the young Chinese female protagonist Yi for Dreamwork's 2019 animated film *Abominable*. Notably, Chloe Benett who is part Chinese and Hailee Stanfield who is part Filpina, were cast in three of these roles; yet their Asian heritage largely has been rendered invisible in the media (Nishime, 2014). Bennet has spoken openly about her decision to change her birth name from Wang to Bennet. She explained, "[c]hanging my last name doesn't change the fact that my BLOOD is half Chinese, that I lived in China, speak Mandarin or that I was culturally raised both American and Chinese. [...] It means I had to pay my rent, and Hollywood is racist and wouldn't cast me with a last name that made them uncomfortable" (Nyren, 2017).

Actor Constance Wu portrayed the only non-youth Asian American lead female characters in the survey of 2007–2019 top-grossing films (Yuen et al., 2021). Wu played one as a highly educated Chinese American professor, Rachel Chu, in the fairytale-like *Crazy Rich Asians* that takes place among an Asian and Asian American cast and is mostly set in Singapore, and the other as Asian American novice stripper Dorothy in the film *Hustlers.* Even though the film more fully and sympathetically develops the character of Dorothy as a woman working with other strip club workers to steal money from their wealthy clients, it is noteworthy that one of the two lead Asian American adult female characters documented by the study still embodies the long-standing stereotype of Asian and Asian American women in the sex industry using their sexuality for manipulative reasons.

Two widely released 2022 films, *Everything Everywhere All at Once* (EEAO) and *Turning Red* (TR), however, indirectly engage broader ideas of gender, health, and the body in groundbreaking ways. Both films reflected the input of Asian American filmmakers and cast members in presenting well-rounded and complex Asian American male and female characters. The first film released by 4D features an immigrant couple Evelyn and Wayland Wong, who run a laundry. Evelyn's perspective as a daughter, wife, and mother is heavily influenced by her dissatisfaction with the economic and social struggle of making in the United States. She is navigating her relationship with her daughter, whose same-sex relationship and inability to live up to the expectations Evelyn faced from her own father and now projects onto her. When Evelyn unexpectedly experiences the different possibilities of her life lived out in different universes, she recognizes how the weight of others' expectations has informed her choices and the expectations she has placed on her family as well. The film's mother-daughter relationship resonates with the mother-daughter relationship in Pixar's *Turning Red,* which is presented through the eyes of the adolescent Asian Canadian Mei. Mei's mother and her maternal line manifest themselves as red pandas, which represent their ancestral heritage. That the red panda shows up when females often begin menses is not a coincidence, conveying the opportunities, possibilities, and dangers the women in Mei's family must confront. Both films explore Asian American women's experiences at different points in the life cycle yet offer similar perspectives about familial expectations and community stereotypes, and how these may be sources of strength and shame alike for Asian American women. The distinction both films make between one's heritage and navigating the conditions of the present (both in North America) also suggests that differences between cultures may be experienced differently across generations of Asian American women. These tensions and differences likewise affect how one understands physical, emotional, and mental health, and how one addresses those specific needs and experiences.

Portrayals of AANHPI women on television unfortunately also reflect the stereotypes and underrepresentation documented in the 2021 study (Yuen et al., 2021). For decades, AANHPI female roles continued to be as extras or with limited speaking roles – as prostitutes, nurses, or villagers in the 1970s television series *MASH* set in Korea or the late 1980s series *China Beach* set in Vietnam. Featured roles for specific stories in the 1980s and 1990s emphasized Asian American females as model minorities, the stereotype that characterized Asian Americans as driven to achieve success in a professional field, either by parental pressure, internal perfectionism, or both: e.g., Ming-Na Wen's role on ER as Chinese American Jing-Mei "Deb" Chen or Kim Miyori's role on *St. Elsewhere* as Japanese American Dr. Wendy Armstrong who was revealed to be bulimic and ultimately committed suicide in the second season.

Increasing numbers of television networks by the 1990s resulted in a few more notable roles: e.g., Japanese American actor Keiko Agina who portrayed a Korean teenager Lane Kim on Warner Brothers' *Gilmore Girls* and Indian American actor Reshma Shetty who played Divya Katdare on USA Network's *Royal Pains.* Like Jing-Mei Chen's character on ER, Reshma Shetty's character also experiences conflicts with her immigrant parents who attempt to control their daughter's life. Thai and Hmong American actor Brenda Song in the early years of 2000 enjoyed a less pigeon-holed role with the Disney Channel's *The Suite Life of Zack of Cody*. In the 21st century, less stereotypical leading roles for adult Asian American female actors – albeit still highly limited – have included Chloe Bennett and Ming-na on *Agents of S.H.I.E.L.D.,* Chinese American Constance Wu on *Fresh Off the Boat,*and Indian American actor Priyanka Chopra (Jonas) on ABC's *Quantico*. Like the U.S. film industry, feature and leading roles for NHPI women have been very rare, with the one exception NBC's *Young Rock*, a comedy about Dwayne "The Rock" Johnson's childhood growing up multiracial with an African American father and Samoan American mother. Stacey Leilua portrays his mother, Ata Johnson, and Ana Tuisila portrays his grandmother Lia Maivia. However, while the greater number of television networks both live and streaming have somewhat increased diversity of portrayals, the larger number of choices for television shows also means more limited exposure of these more diverse portrayals among audiences. The highly limited roles for and portrayals of AANHPI women in the movies still have wider impact in informing how AANHPI women are perceived in U.S. society as foreign, submissive, and hypersexualized. As noted below, the overrepresentation of Asian and Asian American females in online pornography further contributes to these controlling images.

The specific ways Asian women are represented as passive and eager to please as well as hypersexualized also may make AANHPI women targets of sexual violence. Among Asian and Pacific Islander women in the United States, more than one in five AANHPI women had experienced some form of contact sexual violence (23%), and non-contact unwanted sexual experiences (21%) during their lifetime (Smith et al., 2018). One in ten AANHPI women experienced attempted or completed rape (Smith et al., 2018). A 2018 opinion piece in the *New York Times* suggests that White supremacist males are fetishizing Asian and Asian American women as potential partners because of two converging stereotypes: the Cold War model minority myth and the myth of the submissive, hypersexualized Asian woman (Lim, 2018). In other words, model minority as well-behaved, not likely to raise a fuss but simply wanting to fit in by working hard and attaining success is gendered and sexualized. Lim explains that Asian women are "seen as naturally inclined to serve men sexually. … Nowhere is this more explicit than in sex ads and online pornography" (Lim, 2018).

Citing several cases in Canada and the United States where non-Asian males sexually attacked Asian American females, sometimes as serial predators, Park (2012) notes that,

> Asians in the United States, like [I]ndigenous people, but unlike blacks and whites, are most often attacked by non-Asians. … While scholars note that not all of the non-Asian men who desire or are violent towards Asian women are white, all neglect to account for how disparately positioned men perform and sustain white hetero-patriarchal supremacy differently through acts of violence against women (p. 497).

Studies of online rape pornography have found that where the rape victim's race could be identified the majority were young Asian women, and "surmise that Asian women's overrepresentation in internet rape pornography is due to Orientalist representations of Asian females as hyperservile and hypersexual" (Park, 2012, p. 498). Because femininity often is associated with national identities, Park also suggests that violence against Asian females might also provide a way for non-Asian males to assert power in reaction to "Asia's economic ascendancy" in the recent decades (Park, 2012, p. 504).

AANHPI women thus have been racialized, gendered, and sexualized in the United States imagination (Parreñas & Tam, 2008). Their bodies and identities as AANHPI women have been subject to governmental scrutiny via immigration policy. Their experiences as military wives due to U.S. militarization of Asia and the Pacific Islands beginning after World War II subjected them to claims of seeking U.S. citizenship via marriage and seduction, which also continues with stereotypes of AANHPI women as mail order brides. The distinct ways Americans perceive AANHPI women from the beginning of immigration and interaction make a difference for how AANHPI women's sexuality is also perceived in relation to their health.

Accounting for Cultural Health Practices: Challenges to Understanding and Promoting AANHPI Women's Sexual and Reproductive Health

Lisa: For us we have to see a woman doctor 'cause that's our culture. Never see a man.

Joy: Here I have a woman doctor. I don't normally see the men, but I cannot always have [a female doctor.] I'm not open [with the male doctor].

Fran: Yeah. That's why when we first came here ... we felt nervous when we see the doctors, Men doctors. Yeah, we [were] scared and nervous.

-*Conversation among focus group participants*

Asian American women often are ignored when it comes to women's sexual and reproductive health in the United States. Stereotypes about modesty may play a role in how Asian American women are treated as sexual partners. Professor Hyeouk Chris Hahm notes, "This cultural expectation for women to be submissive and accommodating affects her ability to have discussions about HIV Risk and consistent condom use. ... in fact, APIA women who are perceived to have lower relationship power were significantly more likely to be engaged in HIV related risk behaviors" (Veridianio, 2016).

Pacific Islander women likewise have been ignored; the history of U.S. imperialism in the Pacific Islands and the ways that colonization and militarization have affected the economies of the Pacific Islands and motivated migration to the United States for wage work is only part of the story. Growing up in colonized regions with U.S.-trained teachers meant that they were formally taught about sexual and reproductive health through a foreign, Eurocentric lens. Furthermore, the impact of environmental pollution in the Pacific Islands has left a legacy of illness and conditions that have affected sexual and reproductive health.

The lack of attention to AANHPI women's sexual health in general seems particularly striking, given how AANHPI women have been sexualized in both docile and exotic ways (Espiritu, 2004; Hall, 2015). Not surprisingly, the most attention paid to AANHPI women's sexual practices may be in relation to U.S. military bases in Asia and the Pacific beginning in the 1940s. U.S. military base doctors screened prostitutes for sexually transmitted disease and the U.S. military warned personnel to try to avoid intimacies with Asian and Pacific Islander women even as it created programs to prepare war brides for the culture shock of relocating to the United States (Imada, 2012; Parreñas, 2008; Simpson, 2001; Woo, 2019; Yuh, 2002). At the same time, the model minority stereotype that connotes high levels of competency and access to resources, including those related to medical care, may also extend to perceptions of AANHPI health. Growing awareness of AANHPI alternate forms of heath treatment such as acupuncture, cupping, and herbal medicines, may also result in generalizations that equate the use of such methods with heightened health consciousness among the AANHPI communities.

Although most Asian and Pacific Islander cultures openly address sexuality in literature, poetry, and visual imagery, actual discussion of sexuality differs depending on context. Traditional Chinese and Cambodian cultures have limited open discussion about sexuality in the belief that it would discourage premarital sexual activity (Okazaki, 2002). Church and missionary influences in the Pacific Islands, the Philippines, Asia, and among Asian American ethnic enclaves have also contributed to more conservative attitudes toward sexuality, particularly among first generations of immigrants (Okazaki, 2002). Okazaki suggests that cultural factors, including lack of communication with mothers about sexual and reproductive health, modesty about sexuality, fear of disgracing the family, and perceptions of gynecological exams as inappropriate before marriage, may discourage Asian American women from addressing their sexual health. (Okazaki, 2002). A survey of undergraduate Asian American women at a Southern California university found that 55.6% of respondents learned about birth control at school, 45.7% from social sources, 32.1% from healthcare providers, and only 10.8% learned about birth control from family (C. Lee et al., 2013). Asian American parents are more likely to promote abstinence rather than birth control, and tended to believe that sex education was best taught at school (C. Lee et al., 2013). As Heyrana et al. (2023) note, "Asian American adults often avoid preventative sexual and reproductive health care due to language barriers, lack of cultural congruence with health care professionals, limited health literacy, and financial concerns. They are the least likely of all ethnicities to have a personal doctor, undergo routine Pap tests, or obtain mammograms. … Asian American adolescents are less likely to consistently use condoms or other forms of contraception, be knowledgeable about human immunodeficiency virus (HIV) transmission, and feel comfortable disclosing health needs to health care professionals than their White peers" (Heyrana et al., 2023, p. 789).

The array of different factors that affect AANHPI women's own sense of sexuality and sexual confidence have been explored in literature often authored by AANHPI women. The great diversity of AANHPI women – as being recent immigrants (i.e., first-generation) to being fourth or fifth-generation U.S. born; from refugee to work-based migrant, to voluntary immigrant; representing one of over 70 cultural and language groups; to multiple religious affiliations and multiple sexualities or genders; being in different points in the life cycle – result in infinite possible experiences and understandings of one's selfhood and one's sexuality. As Wong and Santa Ana (1999, p. 171) observe,

> … there is no satisfactory … vocabulary for the interconnectedness, mutual constitution, and operational simultaneity of race/ethnicity, gender/ and sexuality. … Mitsuye Yamada deplores the notion that "ethnicity" and "womanhood" are "at war with each other" and resents the pressure on women of color to choose between the two. … Elaine Kim speaks of the "American tangle of race and gender hierarchies" and describes Asian American political and sexual objectification as having been "tightly plaited". … Analyzing Asian women in global capital, Lisa Lowe asserts that "throughout lived social relations, is it apparent that labor is gendered, sexuality is raced, and race is class-associated."

Novels, poems, and short stories provide insights about how AANHPI women navigate inequalities based on sex, socioeconomic status, citizenship status, and cultural expectations from both their ethnic communities as well as U.S. society as part of their everyday lives. Wong and Santa Ana (2004) note that while Asian American women's writings were limited in the early era of Asian migration to the United States (1850s–1950s), women's writings from the 1960s–1980s took place during a time of social movements and cultural change. Anti-imperialism and anti-racism as well as feminist movements informed Asian American women's self-exploration and self-definition in rejecting both Asian and Western forms of patriarchy, "reclaimed sexuality, and declared a new image: tough, powerful, resourceful, independent and courageous" (S.L. C. Wong et al., 1999, pp. 193–194). Maxine Hong Kingston's *The Woman Warrior* and Amy Tan's *Joy Luck Club* featured mother-daughter relationships and were emblematic of the writing during these decades. Other authors "recovered" Asian American women immigrants who endured hardships and created their own lives, providing alternate models of Asian American womanhood (S.L. C. Wong et al., 1999, p. 195).

The dramatic shift in the demographics of Asian America from 1990 onward has resulted in greater attention to diasporic flows and transnational ties, as well as the contributions of Filipinos, Koreans, South Asians, and Southeast Asians in Asian American cultural productions. Wong and Santa Ana (1999) observe that some works detail women confronting colonialism that results in relocating to the United States: "In these works, female sexuality creates a unique vulnerability to colonial or anticolonial, nationalist violence, but it is also a source of strength and the basis of bonds among women" (S.L. C. Wong et al., 1999, p. 201). This period saw greater exploration of father-daughter relationships or makeshift families. The turn of the 21st century also ushered in more writings about "wildness," signaling a resistance to "defining female subjectivity only or primarily in terms of familial and cultural roles" (S.L. C. Wong et al., 1999, pp. 203–204). Greater willingness to address mental illness and sexual violence and abuse is also apparent. Most recently, the aging of transracial adoptees from Asia has also given rise to books about Asian or multiracial Asian daughters navigating their belonging to adoptive families, their adolescence as "outsiders within" White communities, and attempts to reconnect in some way with their Asian heritage. More anthologies of LGBTQ + Asian American first-person narratives have also been published that address multiracial heritage, fictive kinship and navigating Asian norms and expectations (see for example, Doenath & Ramdeen, 2021; Kumashiro, 2004; Manalansan et al., 2021).

Even if fictional, these texts explore the impact these factors have upon AANHPI's self-identity, resilience, and empowerment. Significantly, many novels authored by AANHPI women are written as first-person narratives about women coming into one's sense of self –whether coming of age, acknowledging traumatic events, or learning about one's family history. They share themes of confronting and breaking silences, dissociation, and embodiment, becoming aware of desire and learning how to express it. For example, *Bitter in the Mouth* (Truong, 2011) is a first-person account about growing up in North Carolina, and how an adoptee relates to her adoptive family and a specific regional history that embraces a romance of whiteness. At first read, Linda the narrator is trying to understand the double-edged nature of love as both healing and shattering, and the ways that families reproduce histories across generations. Midway through the novel reveals that Linda is a transracial adoptee who was born in Vietnam and adopted by a White family under mysterious circumstances. Only at the end does the novel reveal that Linda has just been diagnosed with cervical cancer and will not be able to have biological children of her own. What she perceives as her body's betrayal – a body with which she has a fraught relationship – has caused her to ruminate upon what it means to not be able to bear a child, and what it means to not pass down her family bloodline, its mutated genes and history, to another generation.

Several AANHPI authors, along with other women of color, have explored women's embodiment of trauma through silence and muteness, through the merging of the physical and emotional (see for example, Cao, 1997; Duncan, 2009; Keller, 1998; Kingston, 2010). Early trauma theory assumed that traumatic experiences cannot be articulated, but literary scholars have noted how different forms of narration may take the place of physical acts of speaking (Gilmore, 2005, pp. 100–102). Trauma may relentlessly make its way through the body. Linda has synesthesia, a condition that causes her to "taste words," or to associate tastes with the words she hears. However, her sense of detachment from her own history, due to unspoken words about how she came to be adopted, has an even greater impact on her heart. She was stolen from her biological family, loved by her adoptive family, and now, in an emotional state where she cannot discern love from hate nor care from violence, questions what it means to be intimately (dis)connected with others as family.

Kasey: And when you mention cancer being abnormal, like all the diseases that are prevalent within the islands: there's like the cancers, both of, three of my grandparents out of the four have died of cancer and there's diabetes on both sides of the family. There's, I mean, we talk about the pesticides that are in. in things, the hormones – the growth hormones. The chickens are way huger than what we used to grow up with. Talking about the nuclear fallouts that was in the atoll … The Alzheimer's, dementia, there are so many …

Fran: Or the combination of Parkinsons and Alzheimer's. And in Guam for such a small capita we have such a high rate. And even [health researchers have] gone to do research on that. …. And that is super sad.

Kasey: Even birth defects … it's so taboo. I remember not too long ago, they would say, "Oh that's your relative that you don't know about" because they would hide still, because it was shameful to have somebody that's not perfect, right, or not normal. Normal, whatever that is. And now that there's more awareness around different things and even, I remember people used to think that even homosexuality was abnormal and that kind of thing. But know that … it's going to be so empowering to bring awareness toward health and wellness and understanding that we are all going through we are all struggling with the same issues that we can support each other with.

-Conversation among focus group participants

Literature written by NHPI women, on the other hand, often addresses the ongoing colonization of Oceania and the ever-present resistance on the part of Indigenous women. One of the key themes in poetry is a reclamation of language and culture, some of it lost and some it being recovered after the United States forcibly claimed Hawai'i as a territory and then a state. Brandi McDougall, in her extensive discussion about Native Hawaiian poetry (2016), explains the reading practice of "kaona" that reveals meanings just as much as it hides them to ensure the seeker is worthy of finding meaning. Calling readers to engage this knowledge, she quotes from poets Osorio and Wong's "Kaona" (McDougall, 2016, p. 51):

> *With every story forgot,*
> *we lose a piece of our history*
> *It's time to uncover the past that we may understand our future*
> *Interpret our stories that we may better know ourselves*

The impact of foreign influences upon Kānaka Maoli social relations also affected women's roles in society. McDougall (2016) describes Pele and Hi'iaka, goddesses who are central to Kānaka Maoli understandings of their culture, as examples of mana wahine, "a distinctly Indigenous Pacific concept of feminine power and authority" (p. 122). For Kānaka Maoli, mana wahine, is "partially sexual in nature because ... procreation is part of creation, and women give birth to future generations" (p. 124). Other authors address how colonization is reflected in the ongoing influence of U.S. popular culture through television and other media. Sia Figel (1999) describes a Sāmoan teenager entering adulthood in *Where We Once Belonged*; as a young woman growing up in a Sāmoan village, Alofa is influenced by Christianity, *Charlie's Angels*, and U.S. consumer goods, as well as the racism, sexism, and poverty. Alofa's transition to adulthood reflects the indelible imprint of U.S. imperialism's impact on Sāmoa and its effect on her understanding of what it means to be a woman in Sāmoa.

The violence of imperialism in the Pacific Islands also factors into a culture of violence that affects women as well. In 2018, the United Nations estimated that nearly three or four out of five women and girls in the Pacific Islands will experience physical and/or sexual violence in their lifetimes (APIGPV, 2018). Teresia Teaiwa, an I-Kiribati and African American scholar, uses the term "militourism" (1994) to describe how U.S. military bases across the Pacific Islands and Asia are also linked to economic development through tourism in Guåhan and Hawai'i for example. Tourism relies upon marketing Pacific Islander women as sexualized commodities. Teaiwa points out that the bikini evokes images of tropical beaches for tourists but for Pacific Islanders is a reminder of testing of 25 nuclear bombs on Bikini Atoll, a coral reef in the Marshall Islands, between 1946 and 1958 (Teaiwa, 1994). The resulting radioactivity in the environment, particularly the ocean, resulted in cancers and birth defects.

Marshallese poet Kathy Jetñil-Kiljiner describes the effects of the U.S. military conducting nuclear tests on women's reproductive health in her poem "History Project" (Jetñil-Kijiner, 2017, p. 21):

I read first hand accounts of what we call
jelly babies
tiny beings with no bones
skin – red tomatoes
the miscarriages gone unspoken
the broken translations
I never told my husband
I thought it was my fault
I thought
there must be something wrong
inside me

The mutation of nature's reproductive power into devastation extends from the ocean into the food, water, and air, resulting in much higher-than-average birth defects and cancers, interrupting the healthy reproduction of life on the islands. Residents of Bikini Atoll were persuaded to relocate as part of their Christian values. Noting the arrogance of U.S. military personnel, with the general telling elders that the tests are "for the good of mankind" and "God will thank you," Jetñil-Kiljiner's 15-year self, "graph(s) my people's death by cancer and canned food diabetes on flow charts in 3D (p. 7)". Teaiwa proposes the idea of "the s/pacific body" that rejects understanding the physical body as simply biological. She draws upon Black feminist scholar Barbara Christian's point that gender is a social construct, and that the body is *both physical and social* (Teaiwa, 1994, p. 96). NHPI women's sexual health, then, cannot be understood apart from how U.S. colonization and militarization have affected their environments and their health.

The physical and social impacts on the reproductive health and mortality of Pacific Islander women are a political issue as well. The lack of funding for research or oncological care on the Marshallese Islands in the wake of the radiation poisoning resulting from the nuclear bomb tests resulted in no data. The lack of data effectively vanished this issue from public view. In the 1980s, the U.S. government promised the citizens of Compact of Free Association (COFA) nations (the Republic of Palau, Federated States of Micronesia, and the Marshall Islands) the ability to travel freely to the United States and health coverage under Medicaid even though they would not receive U.S. citizenship. In 1996, however, the Personal Workforce Responsibility and Welfare Reform Act, supported by a Democrat president and a Republican House majority, removed COFA citizens from Medicaid coverage. This promise to COFA citizens remained broken until 2023, even as their mortality rate increased by 21% from 2015 to 2018 – a result of the 67 nuclear bombs detonated over the Marshall Islands and lasting effects of radiation (Diamond, 2020). Over 20 years later in 2020, Senator Mazie Hirano (D-HI) led a coalition of congresspeople to pass H.R. 133: Consolidated Appropriations Act. Section 208, which provided Qualified Non-Citizens (QNC) status for anyone from a COFA nation (Hofschneider, 2020) QNC status immediately conferred eligibility for Medicaid retroactive to December 1, 2020. Part of this effort was educating Americans and especially congresspersons about use of the Pacific Islands as experimental sites for nuclear bombs and the disproportionate impact on the bodies and futures of those Pacific Islander communities.

Asian American and Pacific Islander Women's Political Activism

> I'm an immigrant as well but an assimilated Asian immigrant, I am much more vocal about my health issues – I don't minimize them because I feel that often in the Asian community women's health issues aren't necessarily – you know, their aches and pains are just "oh" everyday aches and pains that people complain about as opposed to an underlying cause. And I've noticed that the tendency between my parents of my dad minimizing my mother's health issues to an extent and then we beg him – because they don't live here – to take her to the emergency room and a couple of times she's been hospitalized that way where he's kind of waited. Same thing for my aunt who's kind've complained about her knee problems and headaches and this and this and then turns out that it was something more serious. … and to this day I notice my mother minimizing her health issues and her health things are not taken as seriously. So I'm actually extra vocal about it and I feel like I have to advocate for her.
>
> *-Tess, Focus group participant*

Despite the challenges of lasting harmful stereotypes that make AANHPI women particularly vulnerable to racialized sexual harassment and violence (Park, 2012) and the deterioration of social determinants of health that translates to negative health by "getting under the skin" of AANHPI women over time (Taylor, Repetti, & Seeman, 1997); AANHPI women persist. AANHPI women's activism contributed to raised awareness about AANHPI women's sexual and reproductive health, and efforts towards equity in sexual and reproductive health. AANHPI women were active politically or in asserting their rights as women well before modern feminism. Kānaka Maoli women for example, actively protested the overthrow of the Kingdom of Hawaiʻi that was instigated by U.S.

businessmen who claimed Native Hawaiians could not govern themselves (Silva, 1998). Chinese women in 1874 loudly protested their detention and possible deportation in California's Supreme Court, contesting California's commissioner of immigration's assumption that they were not reuniting with their husbands but were being trafficked as prostitutes and therefore were prohibited entry under California's 1870 Anti-Kidnapping Law (Abrams, 2005). CHamoru scholar DeLisle (2022) documents the ways CHamoru women actively resisted U.S. militarization and intervention in CHamoru's lives early in the 20th century, rejecting U.S. medical personnel and navy wives' attempts to "modernize." She explores the complex interplay of gender, settler colonialism and power in her groundbreaking history about CHamoru pattera (nurse-midwives) and other CHamoru women whose significant cultural labor that accompanied their paid work was a form of resistance against U.S. imperialism in Guåhan (2022).

Amidst the social movements that emerged in the late 1960s and early 1970s, some Asian American women and Pacific Islander women actively asserted their political and social rights in the wake of social movements during the early 1970s, including the Third World internationalist solidarity movement, the Women's Movement, and the Asian American movement. Some Asian American women were inspired by Black radical politics, including the Black Panthers (Wu, 2013) or the Third World Women's Alliance (Hong, 2018). The Black radical critique of U.S. imperialism abroad during the late 1960s and 70s inspired some Asian Americans to work with Black, Indigenous, Puerto Rican, and Latinx women in the interests of anti-imperialist organizations (Hong, 2018). Importantly, these organizations recognized that capitalism was based on the racial exploitation of less developed, formerly colonized nations referred to collectively as Third World nations. Questioning ongoing global disparities in wealth to the ways that non-White communities also faced secondary citizenship and poverty within the United States also informed an analysis of the internal colonization and exploitation of non-White communities within the United States as well. These connections inspired many Americans, particularly non-White Americans, to engage the concept of Third World solidarity across marginalized non-White communities in the United States and with communities in Asia, Africa, and Latin America that had experienced colonization and often were still under neocolonial conditions. Other Asian American women found meaning in the dominant form of feminism, which sought incorporation of women more fully in U.S. society with an emphasis on securing individual rights and opportunities equal to those of men. Patsy Mink, a Japanese American congresswoman from Hawai'i, in fact was the first non-White woman to run for President, and was a major force behind Title IX, the 1972 bill that ensured equality of opportunities for women in higher education (Wu, 2020). As Wu notes, Mink's leadership role demonstrates that liberal feminism was not limited to White, middle-class women. Other AANHPI women activists, like other women of color, explicitly rejected the term feminism because it seemed to only focus on women's equality with men and did not address ongoing struggles of communities of color against racial and economic oppression. Wu's work on the 1977 National Women's Conference in Houston (the only federally funded national conference to address and develop a national platform of women's issues) also documents the participation of Pacific Islander women at this conference. Pacific Islander women – who avoided the term "feminist" because they perceived it as a White-women-led movement for individual rights – participated in the territorial pre-NWC meetings held in American Sāmoa, Guam, and the Trust Territories where differences in policies, politics, and priorities emerged (Wu, 2022). Other scholars recently have also highlighted the NWC participation of African American leaders including Coretta Scott King, Barbara Jordyn, Shirley Chisolm, and Barbara Smith (Giles et al., 2022).

During the 1970s, Native Hawaiian women also actively participated in the Hawaiian Renaissance, a movement among Native Hawaiians to reclaim their culture and history, demilitarize Kānaka Maoli lands, and assert political self-determination. *Nā Wāhine Koa: Hawaiian Women for Sovereignty and Demilitarization* (Akaka et al., 2018) provides the personal stories of four such Kānaka Maoli women activists: Edwina Akaka, Loretta Tiee, Maxina Kahaulaelio and Terrilee Keko'olani-Raymonds, who share their personal stories of lifelong activism of protecting their ancestral lands from desecration by the military, protecting the rights of residents from eviction to make way for development, calling for environmental restoration of the lands, and creating coalitions across Oceania as part of the Nuclear Free and Independent Pacific movement. Even though the women worked with and acknowledge the activism of men as balancing their own, Noelani Goodyear-Ka'ōpua in the introduction observes how historical memory is often gendered. "Namely men are remembered and memorialized more often than women and māhū (transgendered folks)" (Akaka et al., 2018, p. 21). She goes on to suggest that recording the personal stories of these particular women, "is an effort in restoring balance; otherwise, gendered ways of remembering and forgetting will erode the very mountains on which we stand." (*Ibid.,* p. 22).

The activism of other Indigenous Pacific Islander women similarly reflects a commitment to protecting and restoring ancestral lands through environmental movements protesting the impacts of military testing on their islands and ocean waters, participating in anti-militarization movements to end the military presence that negatively affected their island homes and economies, and securing a healthy future for their communities. DeLisle (2022) describes women's activism against increased U.S. militarization of Guåhan during 2017 oversight hearings: “manmaga‘håga (women leaders) reminded federal officials and local leaders of the U.S. military’s historical and ongoing destruction and contamination of the island. They called specific attention to the devastating environmental effects on the southern and northern villages of Santa Rita (near Naval Base Guam) and Yigu (near Andersen Air Force Base), whose residents suffer the highest incidence of cancer and death rates” (DeLisle, 2022, p. 199).

Although AANHPI women initially may have felt caught in between fighting for women’s rights and fighting for community rights, as if they had to choose between prioritizing their rights as women or their communities’ rights (Pegues, 1997), women of color feminist theory articulates the intersection of one’s gender, racial and ethnic identities, sexuality, disability, socioeconomic status, and shared commitments to social justice (Fujiwara & Roshanravan, 2018). In the case of reproductive justice, for example, Pacific Islander communities have seen the impact of environmental pollution on the health of babies being born and on women’s reproductive health; Asian Americans living in urban areas along with other poor, disproportionately non-White, communities, likewise have seen their children’s health negatively affected by asthma and other pollutants (Sze, 2006). Other AANHPI women activists have sought economic justice and better education for their communities, whether these have concentrations of AANHPIs or not; Grace Lee Boggs and Yuri Kochiyama are examples of Asian American activists who were active among the African American neighborhoods in which they lived and created community (Boggs, 2011; Kochiyama et al., 2004) Disability activists continue to raise awareness about the ways in which AANHPI communities themselves can be more inclusive of community members who live with disabilities. Chen observes that the language of rights and freedoms often deployed in activism draws upon ableist metaphors, equating the ability to speak or see with social belonging and rights. She states, “Laura Yung Yi Kang has usefully commented that such attachment to or usage of silence as a disavowed identity has its costs: ‘The repeated rallying cries of ‘breaking silence,’ ‘coming to voice,’ and ‘making visible,’ presuppose some absence, repression, and marginalization …” (Chen, 2013, p. 98). Chen further questions how the inability of “non-English speaking immigrants to the U.S.” also falls within the purview of silence, excluding them yet again from participation in U.S. civic spaces. (Chen, 2013, p. 101).

At the intersection of labor and disability, furthermore, feminist scholars have documented connections between manufacturing and service work and chronic health concerns. Louie’s (2001) documentation of immigrant women workers’ collective organizing and protests to achieve better working conditions also highlights the disabilities that some workers experienced as a result of debilitating working conditions. She writes of Lisa, a first-generation Chinese immigrant who worked in an unregulated subcontractor's sweatshop that paid no overtime and refused days off. "Lisa and her co-workers suffered various injuries and constant fatigue." (p. 19). After being rejected by ILGWU/Unite in the mid-1990s, Lisa and her coworkers were successfully represented by the Chinese Staff and Workers Association of Chinatown in New York City (p. 41). These victories are important, but the chronic pain accompanies workers to new service jobs (p. 37). Kang (2010) researched Korean immigrant women's work in nail salons and reported that almost all of the manicurists described their exposure to toxins as the worst part of their jobs. Noting the harsh fumes and chemicals in the various adhesives and solvents, Kang reports, "Constant handling of these solvents exposes workers to carcinogenic, allergenic, and/or reproductively harmful substances … A 2004 survey of salon employees in New York City revealed that 37% suffered from skin problems, 37% from eye irritations, 57% from allergies, and 66% from neck or back discomfort, and 18%% from asthma." (Kang, 2018, p. 221). Unhealthy work conditions and low wages have inspired women working in low-wage jobs such as garment and electronics manufacturing, as well as nail salons, to organize for their rights. This may include back wages, the right to wear protective gear such as gloves, and lobbying for less toxic chemicals in nail polish, adhesives, and solvents. (Kang, 2010, pp. 226–227).

One contemporary example of the need for AANHPI women to engage politically relates to the ways that Asian culture and Asian women are being depicted in order to limit access to abortions in the United States. According to The National Asian Pacific American Women's Forum (NAPAWF), "thirteen of the fifteen states with the highest Asian American populations have proposed" sex-abortion bans (NAPAWF, 2021, p. 1). Assumptions that Asian Americans will perform abortions to ensure a male child are based on assumptions that sex-selection abortions took place during China's "one-family one-baby law" and infanticide in India (Yeung, 2015) due to those nations' male-biased sex ratios (Citro et al., 2014). Yet European nations with primarily White populations reported higher male-biased sex ratios than either Asian nation (Citro et al., 2014). While a conservative think tank reported in 2011 that birth ratios suggest that foreign-born Chinese, Indians, and Koreans have been performing sex-selective abortions, analysis of the single study cited to support this claim (Almond and Edlund) and subsequent research demonstrated families from these three Asian ethnic groups "have *more* girls on average than whites" (Citro et al., 2014, p. 16). These bans would require abortion providers to ensure that people seeking abortions are not doing so because of the fetus's sex. As NAPAWF notes, "These stereotypes about the values of AANHPI communities are not only ugly – they are dangerous, inaccurate, and encourage racial profiling in health care" (NAPAWF, 2021, p. 1). These laws resonate with the 1875 Page Law, a federal law that denied Chinese women entry to the United States based on immigration officials' assumptions that most Chinese women were entering for purposes of prostitution, not to reunite with their husbands. This continual national scrutiny of AANHPI women's bodies and motivations based on dominant gendered and racial stereotypes speaks to ongoing needs for Asian American, Native Hawaiian, and Pacific Islander women to be aware of the ways they are positioned not only in relation to each other, but to other women (particularly other women of color) as well to define who belongs in U.S. society and who does not.

Feminist of color disability studies further emphasize understanding the importance of women being able to make their own decisions about their own bodies, reminding us that those challenges confronting women locally are shared by women around the world. As Erevelles has observed, governments worldwide have enacted policies and laws that limit citizenship, reproduction, and economic health for women who do not fit their definition of who belongs – whether this be because of poverty, immigration status, disability, or race/ethnicity (Erevelles, 2011). Schalk and Kim further note, "nationalist discourses of (dis) ability shape not only immigration laws, such as the Chinese Exclusion Act of 1882 … but also the treatment of immigrants, people read as immigrants (that is, people of color, especially those with English as a second language), and other groups, such as disabled and poor people who are considered burdens on the financial health of the nation (Stanley et al., 2013, p. 77)" (Schalk & Kim, 2020, p. 41). We see this in the experiences of AANHPI women whose histories are indeed transnational, spanning the U.S., Hawai'i, the Pacific Islands, and Asia.

References

Abrams, K. (2005). Polygamy, prostitution, and the federalization of immigration law. *Columbia Law Review*, *105*(3), 641–716.

Akaka, M., Kahaulelio, M., Kekoolani-R., T., Ritte, L., & Goodyear-Kaōpua, N. E. (2018). *Nā Wāhine Koa: Hawaiian Women for sovereignty and demilitarization*. University of Hawaii Press.

Asian Pacific Institute on Gender-Based Violence (APIGBV), (2018). *Fact Sheet: Pacific Islanders and Domestic & Sexual Violence*. Retrieved from Asian Pacific Institute on Gender-Based Violence: aapidata.com/wp-content/uploads/2019/03/DVFactSheet-Pacific-Islander-Apr-2018-formatted-2019.pdf

Bailey, B. L., & Farber, D. (1994). *The first strange place: Race and sex in World War II Hawaii*. New York, NY: JHU Press.
Boggs, G. L., & Kurashige, S. (2011). *The next American revolution: Sustainable activism for the twenty-first century*. University of California Press.
Budiman, A. & Ruiz, N.G. (2021). *Asian Americans are the fastest growing ethnic group in the U.S. Pew Research Center*. Retrieved from https://www.pewresearch.org/short-reads/2021/04/09/asian-americans-are-the-fastest-growing-racial-or-ethnic-group-in-the-u-s/
Cao, L. (1997). *Monkey bridge*. New York, NY: Viking Press.
Chan, S. (1991a). *Asian Americans: An interpretive history*. Boston: Twayne Publishers.
Chan, S. (1991b). *Entry denied: Exclusion and the Chinese community in America, 1882–1943*. Philadelphia: Temple University Press.
Chen, M. Y. (2013). Asian American speech, civic place, and future nondisabled bodies. *Amerasia Journal, 39*(1), 91–106. 10.17953/amer.39.1.n6t6477372245h46
Choi, S. K. (2021). *Black LGBT adults in the US: LGBT well-being at the intersection of race*. Williams Institute, UCLA School of Law.
Citro, B., Gilson, J., Kalantry, S., & Stricker, K. (2014). *Replacing myths with facts: Sex-selective abortion laws in the United States*. Retrieved from https://scholarship.law.cornell.edu/facpub/1399/
Crenshaw, K. (2021). Demarginalizing the intersection of race and sex: A black feminist critique of antidiscrimination doctrine, feminist theory and antiracist politics. *Droit et société, 108*, 465.
DeLisle, C. T. (2022). *Placental politics: CHamoru women, white womanhood, and Indigeneity under US colonialism in Guam*. UNC Press Books.
Desmond, J. C. (1997). Invoking "The Native": Body politics in contemporary Hawaiian tourist shows. *The Tulane Drama Review, 41*(4), 83–109. doi:10.2307/1146662
Diamond, D. (2020). 'They did not realize we are human beings,' *Politico*. Retrieved from https://www.politico.com/news/magazine/2020/01/26/marshall-islands-iowa-medicaid-103940
Doenath, G., & Ramdeen, K. (2021). *Untold: Defining moments of the uprooted*. Mango & Marigold Press.
Duncan, P. (2009). *Tell this silence: Asian American women writers and the politics of speech*. University of Iowa Press.
Erevelles, N. (2011). *Disability and difference in global contexts: Enabling a transformative body politic*. Springer.
Espiritu, Y. L. (1993). *Asian American panethnicity: Bridging institutions and identities*. Temple University Press.
Espiritu, Y. L. (1997). *Asian American women and men: Labor, laws, and love*. Rowman & Littlefield.
Espiritu, Y. L. (2004). Asian American panethnicity: Contemporary national and transnational possibilities. In N. Foner & G. M. Fredrickson (Eds.), *Not Just Black and White: Historical and Contemporary Perspectives on Immigration, Race, and Ethnicity in the United States*, 217–234. Russell Sage Foundation.
Figiel, S. (1999). *Where we once belonged*. Kaya Press.
Fojas, C. (2014). *Islands of empire: Pop culture and US power*. University of Texas Press.
Fujiwara, L., & Roshanravan, S. (Eds.). (2018). *Asian American feminisms and women of color politics*. University of Washington Press.
Giles, K.N., Daniel, R.J., & Lovett, L.L. (2022). *It's our movement now: Black women's politics and the 1977 National Women's Conference*. University Press of Florida.
Gilmore, L. (2005). *Autobiography's wounds*. Rutgers University Press.

Goodyear-Kaōpua, N., Hussey, I., & Wright, E. K. (2014). *A nation rising: Hawaiian movements for life, land, and sovereignty*. Duke University Press.
Hall, L. K. (2015). Which of these things is not like the other: Hawaiians and other Pacific Islanders are not Asian Americans, and all Pacific Islanders are not Hawaiian. *American Quarterly*, *67*(3), 727–747. doi:https://www.jstor.org/stable/43823232
Heyrana, K. J., Kaneshiro, B., Soon, R., Nguyen, B. T., & Natavio, M. F. (2023). Data equity for Asian American and Native Hawaiian and other Pacific Islander people in reproductive health research. *Obstetrics & Gynecology*, *142*(4), 787–794. doi:10.1097/AOG.0000000000005340
Hing, B. O. (1993). *Making and remaking Asian America: 1850-1990* (Vol. 74). Stanford University Press.
Hofschneider, A. (2020). How decades of advocacy helped restore Medicaid access to Micronesian migrants. *Honolulu Civil Beat*. Retrieved from https://www.civilbeat.org/2020/12/how-decades-of-advocacy-helped-restore-medicaid-access-to-micronesian-migrants/
Hollinger, D. A. (2006). *Postethnic America: Beyond multiculturalism*. Hachette UK.
Hong, G. K. (2018). Intersectionality and incommensurability. In L. Fujiwara & S. Roshanravan (Eds.), *Asian American Feminisms and Women of Color Politics*. University of Washington Press, 27–42.
Imada, A. L. (2012). *Aloha America: Hula circuits through the US empire*. Duke University Press.
Jetñil-Kijiner, K. (2017). *Iep jaltok: Poems from a Marshallese daughter* (Vol. 80). University of Arizona Press.
Kaholokula, J. K., Okamoto, S. K., & Yee, B. W. (2019). Special issue introduction: Advancing Native Hawaiian and other Pacific Islander health. *Asian American Journal of Psychology*, *10*(3), 197–205. doi:10.1037/aap0000167
Kang, M. (2010). *The managed hand: Race, gender, and the body in beauty service work*. University of California Press.
Kang, M. (2020). Reproducing Asian American studies: Rethinking Asian exclusion as reproductive exclusion. *Amerasia Journal*, *46*(2), 136–146. doi:10.1080/00447471.2020.1840319
Keller, N. O. (1998). *Comfort woman*. Penguin.
Kingston, M. H. (2010). *The woman warrior: Memoirs of a girlhood among ghosts*. Vintage.
Kochiyama, Y., Lee, M., Kochiyama-Sardinha, A., & Kochiyama-Holman, A. (2004). *Passing it on: A memoir*. UCLA Asian American Studies Center Press.
Konzett, D. C. (2017). *Hollywood's Hawaii: Race, nation, and war*. Rutgers University Press.
Kumashiro, K. K. (2004). *Restoried selves: Autobiographies of queer Asian-Pacific-American activists*: Psychology Press.
Lee, C., Tran, D. Y., Thoi, D., Chang, M., Wu, L., & Trieu, S. L. (2013). Sex education among Asian American college females: Who is teaching them and what is being taught. *Journal of Immigrant and Minority Health*, *15*, 350–356. doi:10.1007/s10903-012-9668-5
Lee, J., & Ramakrishnan, K. (2020). Who counts as Asian. *Ethnic and Racial Studies*, *43*(10), 1733–1756. doi:10.1080/01419870.2019.1671600
Leong, K. J. (2001). "A Distinct and Antagonistic Race": Constructions of Chinese manhood in the exclusionist debates, 1869–1878. In M. Basso, L. McCall, & D. Garceau (Eds.), *Across the Great Divide* (pp. 131–148). Routledge.

Lim, A. (2018). The Alt-Right's Asian Fetish. *New York Times*. Retrieved from https://www.nytimes.com/2018/01/06/opinion/sunday/alt-right-asian-fetish.html

Louie, M. C. Y. (2001). *Sweatshop warriors: Immigrant women workers take on the global factory*. South End Press.

Loyd, J. M., Mitchell-Eaton, E., & Mountz, A. (2016). The militarization of islands and migration: Tracing human mobility through US bases in the Caribbean and the Pacific. *Political Geography*, *53*, 65–75. doi:10.1016/j.polgeo.2015.11.006

Manalansan, M., Hom, A. Y., Fajardo, K. B., & Eng, D. L. (2021). *Q&A: Voices from queer Asian North America* (Vol. 231). Temple University Press.

Marchetti, G. (1994). *Romance and the yellow peril: Race, sex, and discursive strategies in Hollywood fiction*. University of California Press.

McDougall, B. N. (2016). *Finding meaning: Kaona and contemporary Hawaiian literature*. University of Arizona Press.

McGregor, D. P. (2003). Constructed images of Native Hawaiian women. In *Asian/Pacific Islander American Women* (pp. 23–41). New York University Press.

Moon, K. H. (1997). *Sex among allies: Military prostitution in US-Korea relations*: Columbia University Press.

NAPAWF. (2021). *Sex-selective abortion ban fact sheet*. Retrieved from https://static1.squarespace.com/static/5ad64e52ec4eb7f94e7bd82d/t/5ffc71263e84173251a59c31/1610379558892/ssab-factsheet-jan-11-2021.pdf

Nishime, L. (2014). *Undercover Asian: Multiracial Asian Americans in visual culture*. University of Illinois Press.

Niumeitolu, F. (2015). *Pacific Islanders march for self determination*. Retrieved from https://morethantwominutes.wordpress.com/2015/03/02/pacific-islanders-march-for-self-determination/

Nyren, E. (2017). 'Agents of SHIELD' star says she changed her last name because 'Hollywood is Racist'. Retrieved from https://variety.com/2017/tv/news/chloe-bennet-last-name-change-hollywood-racism-1202544188/

Okazaki, S. (2002). Influences of culture on Asian Americans' sexuality. *Journal of Sex Research*, *39*(1), 34–41. doi:http://www.jstor.org/stable/3813421

Omi, M., & Winant, H. (1994). *Racial formation in the United States: From the 1960s to the 1990s*. Routledge.

Pacheco, A. M. K. (2010). Past, present, and politics: A look at the Hawaiian sovereignty movement. *Intersections*, *10*(1), 341–387.

Park, H. (2012). Interracial violence, western racialized masculinities, and the geopolitics of violence against women. *Social & Legal Studies*, *21*(4), 491–509. doi:10.1177/0964663912443919

Parreñas, R. S. (2008). *The force of domesticity: Filipina migrants and globalization*. NYU Press.

Parreñas, R. S., & Tam, W. (2008). The derivative status of Asian American women. *In R.S. Parreñas, The force of domesticity: Filipina migrants and globalization*, 110–135. doi:10.18574/nyu/9780814768556.003.0009

Pegues, J. (1997). Strategies from the field: Organizing the Asian American feminist movement. In S. Shah (Ed.) *Dragon ladies: Asian-American Feminists Breathe Fire*, 3–16. South End Press.

Salinas, J. (2020). *What shaped their views on self-determination?* Retrieved from https://www.pacificislandtimes.com/post/2020/10/23/what-shaped-their-views-on-self-determination

Sasa, S. M., & Yellow Horse, A. J. (2022). Just data representation for Native Hawaiians and Pacific Islanders: A critical review of systemic Indigenous erasure in census and recommendations for psychologists. *American Journal of Community Psychology*, *69*(3-4), 343–354. doi:10.1002/ajcp.12569

Schalk, S., & Kim, J. B. (2020). Integrating race, transforming feminist disability studies. *Signs: Journal of Women in Culture and Society*, *46*(1), 31–55. doi:10.1086/718866

Shimizu, C. P. (2007). *The hypersexuality of race: Performing Asian/American women on screen and scene*. Duke University Press.

Silva, N. K. (1998). Kanaka Maoli resistance to annexation. *Oiwi: A Native Hawaiian Journal*, *1*(1), 40–75.

Silva, N. K. (2004). *Aloha betrayed: Native Hawaiian resistance to American colonialism*. Duke University Press.

Simpson, C. C. (2001). *An absent presence: Japanese Americans in postwar American culture, 1945–1960*. Duke University Press.

Smith, S. G., Zhang, X., Basile, K. C., Merrick, M. T., Wang, J., Kresnow, M.-j., & Chen, J. (2018). The national intimate partner and sexual violence survey: 2015 data brief–updated release.

Stanley, S. K., Buenavista, T., Masequesmay, G., & Uba, L. (2013). Enabling conversations: Critical pedagogy and the intersections of race and disability studies. *Amerasia Journal*, *39*(1), 75–82.

Sze, J. (2006). *Noxious New York: The racial politics of urban health and environmental justice*. MIT press.

Taylor, S. E., Repetti, R. L., & Seeman, T. (1997). Health psychology: What is an unhealthy environment and how does it get under the skin? *Annual review of psychology*, *48*(1), 411–447. doi:10.1146/annurev.psych.48.1.411

Teaiwa, T. K. (1994). bikinis and other s/pacific n/oceans. *The Contemporary Pacific*, 87–109.

Truong, M. (2011). *Bitter in the Mouth: A Novel*. Random House Trade Paperbacks.

U. S. Census Bureau. (2019). 2015-2019 American community survey 5-year estimates; generated by Aggie J. Yellow Horse; using American Factfinder; http://factfinder2.census.gov.

Veridianio, R. (2016). Little Sex Ed, Stereotypes Could Lead to Health Risks, Family Planning Issues. *NBC News*. Retrieved from https://www.nbcnews.com/news/asia-america/little-early-sex-ed-sterotyping-could-lead-health-risks-family-n586611

Wong, M. M., Klingle, R. S., & Price, R. K. (2004). Alcohol, tobacco, and other drug use among Asian American and Pacific Islander adolescents in California and Hawaii. *Addictive Behaviors*, *29*(1), 127–141. doi:10.1016/S0306-4603(03)00079-0

Wong, S.L. C., & Santa Ana, J. J. (1999). Gender and sexuality in Asian American literature. *Signs: Journal of Women in Culture and Society*, *25*(1), 171–226. doi:10.1086/495418

Woo, S. (2019). *Framed by War: Korean children and women at the crossroads of U.S. empire*. New York University Press.

Wu, J.T.-C. (2013). *Radicals on the road: internationalsim, orientalism, and feminism during the Vietnam Era*. Cornell University Press.

Wu, J. T.-C. (2020). Asian American feminisms and legislative activism: Patsy Takemoto Mink in the US Congress. In S. Hune & G. Nomura (Eds.), *Our Voices, Our Histories* (pp. 304–320). New York University Press.

Wu, J. T.-C. (2022). Pacific feminist imaginaries: The 1977 US National Women's Conference and the politics of territorial representation. *Transatlantica*, *1*(1). 10.4000/transatlantica.18515

Yamamoto, T. (1999). *Masking selves, making subjects: Japanese American women, identity, and the body*. University of California Press.

Yeung, M. (2015). How Asian American women became the target of anti-abortion activism. *Washington Post*. Retrieved from https://www.washingtonpost.com/posteverything/wp/2015/11/04/how-asian-american-women-became-the-target-of-anti-abortion-activism/

Yuen, N. W., Smith, S. L., Pieper, K., Choueiti, M., Yao, K., & Dinh, D. (2021). The prevalence and portrayal of Asian and Pacific Islanders across 1,300 popular films. *USC Annenberg Inclusion Initiative*. https://assets.uscannenberg.org/docs/aii_aapi-representation-across-films-2021-05-18.pdf

Yuh, J.-Y. (2002). *Beyond the shadow of camptown: Korean military brides in America* New York University Press.

Zhou, M., & Lee, J. (2017). Hyper-selectivity and the remaking of culture: Understanding the Asian American achievement paradox. *Asian American Journal of Psychology*, *8*(1), 7–15. doi:https://psycnet.apa.org/doi/10.1037/aap0000069

Zia, H. (2000). *Asian American dreams: The emergence of an American people*. Farrar, Straus, & Giroux.

2 Just Representation in Data: Data Disaggregation and Asian American, Native Hawaiian, and Pacific Islander Women's Sexual and Reproductive Health

How Asian American, Native Hawaiian and Pacific Islander peoples and communities are represented in data can have important real-life implications. Being meaningfully represented in data means that data captures the realities of peoples, and this information can be used to assess and improve their lives. Representation in federal data – including the national Census every ten years – is particularly important as it is often related directly to distributive justice (i.e., equitable distribution of resources) (Rowse, 2012) and because this data influences how government funding is allocated for American communities. Population data provided by the federal census is used to map the boundaries of voting districts, which are the basis from which representatives for school boards, state legislators, and members of the U.S. House of Representatives are elected. This process of redefining a state's voting districts is called redistricting. In addition, Census data is also used by the federal government to distribute billions of dollars to fund community infrastructure (e.g., roads and hospitals) as well as social programs (e.g., school lunch programs) (U.S. Census Bureau, 2020). Put differently, adequate and just representation in data is not only related to recognition (Arfken, 2013) but also to ensuring equitable distribution of resources (Nobles, 2000) for our communities that are linked to the health of the Asian American, Native Hawaiian, and Pacific Islander peoples and communities.

AANHPI Categorization, Population Changes and Representation in Data

How Asian American, Native Hawaiian and Pacific Islander peoples and communities are represented in data is closely tied to how different groups are categorized. Because some AANHPI ethnicities are numerically small populations, too small to make statistical differences, complex issues contribute to invisibility of AANHPI persons and communities in data. One issue that contributes to such lack of visibility is racial categorization

DOI: 10.4324/9781003449867-3

used in the collection and usage of data. Asian American as a panethnic group identity refers to both the *achieved* self-identity based on collective struggles during the Civil Rights era (Espiritu, 1993; Okamoto, 2003, 2014; Zia, 2000), and the *ascribed* identity through racialization (i.e., a socio-historical process by which race is socially constructed) (Omi & Winant, 1994). In comparison, the aggregated category of "AANHPI" is an *imposed* category that came from the classification of race and ethnicity in federal data by the U.S. government (Humes & Hogan, 2009). The use of such an imposed category raises an important question for AANHPI communities and in our collective work towards advocating for health equity about whether using the federal categorization of our communities can be an effective tool in achieving our goals (Cokley & Awad, 2013).

Inclusion of Asian Americans in U.S. Census data collection first began in the 1870 Census where the "Chinese" category was included as one of the options in addition to four other categories: "White," "Black," "Mulatto," and "Indian" (referring to American Indian or Alaska Native"). The "Japanese" category was added in the 1890 Census; followed by inclusion of the "Filipino," "Korean," and "Hindu" (referring to South Asians regardless of religion) in the 1920 Census (Pew Research Center, 2020). These inclusions of multiple Asian ethnic categories did not stay consistent nor exclusive until the 1990 Census. Similarly, the first time the "Hawaiian" category was included was in the 1960 Census. Then, the "Samoan" and "Guamanian" categories were added in the 1980 Census. The first official category used to categorize AANHPI individuals and communities into one aggregated category, "Asian and Pacific Islander," began in the 1980s (U.S. OMB, 1997). However, Asian Americans and Pacific Islanders who did not belong to the included nine categories (i.e., Chinese, Japanese, Filipino, Korean, Asian Indian, Vietnamese, Hawaiian, Sāmoan, and Guamanian) were categorized as "Others" with other racial and multiracial peoples.

The aggregated "Asian and Pacific Islander" categorization initially was intended to include all individuals coming from countries in Asia and the Pacific due to the small population sizes of each group that falls under this "catch all" category. However, as we explored in the previous chapter, the AANHPI population has been experiencing an incredible population growth since the Immigration and Nationality Act of 1965 which removed the racial quota enacted in 1924 (Lee, 2015, 2019). The AANHPI population grew from less than 0.5% of the total U.S. population in 1960 to 5.7% of the total U.S. population in 2019 – a span of less than 60 years. It is important to emphasize that this population growth also accompanied growing diversity within the AANHPI population, which made the "Asian and Pacific Islander" category even more problematic. For example, in 1960, only three Asian ethnic groups and no Pacific Islander groups were represented in the Census (i.e., Japanese, Chinese and Filipino) (U.S. Census Bureau, 1960).[1] In 2019, 21 distinct Asian ethnic groups and six distinct Pacific Islander groups were represented (i.e., Native Hawaiian, Sāmoan, Tongan, Guamanian or CHamoru, Marshallese and Fijian) (U.S. Census Bureau, 2019). In addition, post-1965 Asian immigrants – on average – have higher educational attainment and socioeconomic status due to policies that targeted highly educated and professional immigrants (Tran et al., 2018; Zhou & Lee, 2017).

These factors together have contributed to significant diversity within the AANHPI community. In fact, Asian Americans had the largest within-group income inequality in the United States in 2016 (Kochhar & Cilluffo, 2018). For example, when the ratio of income at the 90th percentile to income at the 10th percentile within U.S. racial and ethnic groups was assessed, Asian Americans in the top 10 percentile earned nearly 10.7 times more than Asian Americans in the bottom 10 percentile (Kochhar & Cilluffo, 2018). This is the highest within-group difference compared to Black Americans (9.8), non-Latinx White Americans (7.8) and Latinx/Hispanic Americans (7.8) (Kochhar & Cilluffo, 2018). Similar significant group differences within the Asian American panethnic group can be observed when we think about the differences in median annual household income across different Asian ethnic groups.[2] Median household income is the number that is in the middle of the range of household income among a given group, with an equal amount of numbers below and above. In 2015, the median household income for all Asian Americans was $73,060 compared to $53,600 among all U.S. households (López et al., 2017). Yet, the median household incomes were significantly higher for some Asian groups including Indian Americans ($100,000), Filipinos ($80,000) and Japanese ($74,000) (López et al., 2017). At the same time, many Asian groups have significantly lower median household incomes: Burmese ($36,000), Nepalese ($43,500), Hmong ($48,000) and Bangladeshi ($49,800) (López et al., 2017). Available data show substantial group differences between Asian Americans and Pacific Islanders as well. For example, in 2019, per capita income for Asian Americans was $40,524 whereas it was $24,961 for Pacific Islanders; Pacific Islanders had a higher proportion of the population who had income below the poverty level (17.5%) than Asian Americans (10.9%) (U.S. Census Bureau, 2019).

As the fastest growing racial and ethnic minority group in the United States since 2000 and the only racialized group whose population growth is driven by immigration[3] (López et al., 2017), the diversity within the AANHPI community will grow even more significantly over time. Population projections from the Pew Research Center illustrate that immigration will continue to be a significant contributor to changes in population characteristics as the share of the U.S. population that is foreign born is expected to increase from 14% in 2015 to 18% in 2016 (Cohn, 2015). By 2065, the Asian American population is expected to grow from making up about 6% of the U.S. population to 14%, largely driven by international migration. Furthermore, the increasing emigration in the Pacific region due to climate change (Locke, 2009) – as well as the continuing dispossession and displacement of Pacific Islanders (Sasa et al., 2022) – will likely lead to the increase of Pacific Islander migration to the U.S. mainland and immigration to the United States.

Two-Level Data Disaggregation is Critical for AANHPI Communities

The current and increasing diversity within the AANHPI umbrella category makes our ability to understand different communities within the AANHPI category even more urgent. While there are important implications for being able to advocate for our communities as the AANHPI panethnic group, including being represented in data collection and policy dialogues, we must be cautious about how such aggregation may mask significant and meaningful differences within our communities. In particular, we must be able to have access to data that can be disaggregated – separated out – by country of origin and other important factors (e.g., immigration cohort, citizenship/legal status, etc.). Data disaggregation must occur at two levels for AANHPI communities at minimum. First, we must be able to look at the group differences between Asian Americans and Pacific Islanders within the AANHPI category. Second, we must be able to look at within group differences for both Asian Americans and Pacific Islanders (e.g., Korean Americans vs. Hmong Americans; Native Hawaiians vs. Marshallese).

First, the ability to disaggregate the AANHPI category into two subcategories of Asian Americans and Pacific Islanders is important. We will call this the ***first-level data disaggregation***. This effort for the first-level data disaggregation is important because Pacific Islanders have different histories and relations with the U.S. government through their experiences of U.S. imperialism and settler colonialism compared to Asian Americans (Tiongson Jr, 2019). Consequently, disaggregating Pacific Islanders from Asian Americans allows us to look at how U.S. settler colonialism is linked to health inequities of Pacific Islanders. Furthermore, this is especially important for understanding the relationships between Asian American and Pacific Islander communities. As settlers who are occupying Indigenous lands in the United States – especially Asian settlers in Hawai`i, there are important differences in how Asian Americans and Pacific Islanders are impacted by the lasting legacies of U.S. settler colonialism, including its impacts on health (Tiongson Jr, 2019).

This effort for the first-level data disaggregation is partially in place. As mentioned earlier, the emergence of the AANHPI category came from the federal government's creation and use of the "Asian and Pacific Islander" in the 1980s (U.S. Census Budget, 1997; Humes & Hogan, 2009). After decades of community activism to separate Pacific Islanders from Asian Americans, the U.S. Office of Management and Budget finally revised the "standards" for race classification in federal data in 1997 (U.S. OMB Budget, 1997). This new standard separated Pacific Islanders from the "AANHPI" category, created their own category, "Native Hawaiian and Other Pacific Islanders" (NHOPI) (U.S. OMB Budget, 1997). However, despite this change of standard in 1997, the federal government and different health institutions predominantly continue to use the AANHPI category (Kaholokula et al., 2019; Panapasa et al., 2011). Such lack of the first-level data disaggregation in practice leads to inadequate and unjust representation of Pacific Islanders in data (Sasa & Yellow Horse, 2022).

Second, we also need the ability to disaggregate further within the Asian American category and Pacific Islander category by key indicators of difference, mainly country of origin. We will call this the ***second-level data disaggregation***. Within each panethnic category, there still exists substantial diversity as different subgroups from multiple countries of origin all have their unique push and pull factors that led to immigration with their own historical and sociopolitical contexts. For example, Japanese Americans began arriving in the 19th century (Lee, 2015), and only about 27% of Japanese Americans today are foreign born (López et al., 2017). In contrast, nearly 92% of Bhutanese Americans are foreign born as many recently arrived in the United States as refugees after the 1990s (López et al., 2017). As mentioned earlier, there is a great deal of variability in socioeconomic status by subgroups within the Asian American category; aggregation masks important differences and different needs. Specifically, the advantageous characteristics of some subgroups "cancel out" the relatively disadvantageous characteristics of other subgroups in aggregation (Noah, 2018).

Similarly, there are important differences within the aggregated Pacific Islander category (Kaholokula et al., 2019; Spickard et al., 2002). For example, some Pacific Islanders from the U.S. Territories of Guam and the Commonwealth of the Northern Mariana Islands are considered U.S. citizens with access to federal- and state-funded services. At the same time, Pacific Islanders from the Freely Associated States (i.e., the Federated States of Micronesia, the Republic of the Marshall Islands, and the Republic of Palau) are not U.S. citizens (Kaholokula et al., 2019; Spickard et al., 2002). As noted earlier, this has led to substantive differences in access to health care services.

Data Disaggregation for Health Equity of AANHPI Peoples and Communities

Adequate and just representation of AANHPI peoples is also a key part of being able to fully and meaningfully understand AANHPI women's health. That is, being able to understand the current status of health for AANHPI populations is the first critical step to further imagine the efforts to work towards reducing and eliminating health inequalities. Currently, national-level surveys (e.g., National Health Interview Survey) are used to generate the population health estimates that are used as the benchmarks for the population's health. This approach is intended to understand and address the specific needs of different communities in the United States, but obtaining accurate and valid estimates for numerically small populations is extremely difficult with the survey approach.

Compared to lack of adequate representation in federal population data (e.g., U.S. Census data) discussed above, ensuring adequate representation in survey data is accompanied by additional challenges. Given the cultural and linguistic diversity and translation needs within the AANHPI aggregated category, it becomes extremely expensive to include a large enough number of sampled AANHPI individuals in the survey and national surveys often only include a few ethnic groups. Even when appropriate surveys and efforts are in place, AANHPI peoples may not have a high response rate. Research shows that there are high levels of distrust in the government and its data collection among AANHPI people and communities. For example, both Asian Americans and Pacific Islanders reported high levels of opposition to participating in the Census according to the 2020 Census Barriers, Attitudes, and Motivators Survey (CBAMS) (McGeeney et al., 2019). Asian Americans reported the highest fear of repercussions where nearly 41% of Asian Americans indicated high levels of concerns that the Census could be used against them (compared to only 16% of non-Hispanic/Latinx White individuals) (McGeeney et al., 2019). Similarly, nearly 63% of Pacific Islanders[4] reported that they do not trust the federal government "to do what is right" (McGeeney et al., 2019). Such high levels of distrust (i.e., what March & Dibben (2005) term "highest level of negative trust"[5] are not unfounded and are justified in that such distrust comes from complex histories of systemic abuse and exploitation of AANHPI people and communities by the U.S. government. The systemic abuse and exploitation include but are not limited to systemic erasure of Pacific Islanders in data through dispossession and displacement of Pacific Islanders (Sasa & Yellow Horse, 2022), as well as the illegal use of Census data as a roster for Japanese incarceration during the World War II (Seltzer & Anderson, 2007). As a result, AANHPI populations often are not adequately represented in national surveys. Such inadequate AANHPI presentation in data means that AANHPI communities do not have access to information about their own communities, and lack of information translates to AANHPI communities not receiving needed federal funding.

While adequate representation of AANHPI peoples and communities in data remains challenging, the need for data aggregation for the AANHPI peoples and communities is especially critical for advocating for and promoting health equity and health justice. Just as demographic population characteristics (e.g., percentage of the population who are foreign born) and socioeconomic characteristics differ within and across groups within the AANHPI aggregated category, there exist substantial and meaningful differences in nearly all health profiles and key determinants of health (i.e., individual behaviors, medical care, social and physical environments) (Kindig et al., 2008). For example, even at the first level of disaggregation (i.e., disaggregating "Asian Americans" and "Pacific Islanders"), we can observe important differences. Compared to Asian Americans, research documents the profound health inequities Native Hawaiian and Pacific Islanders experience with disproportionately higher rates of worse health outcomes, including chronic physical conditions (e.g., heart diseases and diabetes) (Bitton et al., 2010; Kaholokula et al., 2019; Mau et al., 2009), mental health conditions (e.g., depression) (Hooker et al., 2019), and behavioral health concerns (Wong et al., 2004). Pacific Islanders are also less likely to have access to health care (Bitton et al., 2010), and are more likely to be exposed to worse social and physical environments (Young et al., 2018).

The need for data aggregation for the AANHPI community is certainly not a new issue. Scholars and activists have been advocating for data disaggregation in health data for multiple decades (Mays et al., 2003; Nguyen, Nguyen, & Nguyen, 2013; Srinivasan & Guillermo, 2000; Taualii et al., 2011; Teranishi et al., 2014). The "Asian American and Pacific Islander data disaggregation movement" is an ongoing collaborative effort among academics, community activists and community members for systemic policy change in data collection and representation (Teranishi et al., 2014). These collaborations have already brought important advancements towards meaningful data disaggregation. For example, the Centers for Disease Control and Prevention (CDC) collected the first ever Native Hawaiian and Pacific Islander National Health Interview Survey (NHPI NHIS) in 2015 as the result of community advocacy from Asian American, Kānaka Maoli, and Pacific Islander communities (Panapasa et al., 2011; Wu & Bakos, 2017).

The NHPI NHIS is an unprecedented nationally representative survey that collected information from about 3,000 Native Hawaiian and Pacific Islander households from all 50 states (Panapasa et al., 2011; CDC, 2017; Wu & Bakos, 2017). This data allows meaningful data disaggregation to not only look at health of Native Hawaiians and Pacific Islanders as an aggregated racialized group (i.e., the first-level disaggregation), but also within group differences (e.g., Sāmoans vs. Marshallese) (i.e., the second-level disaggregation). Findings from the data have been instrumental in having more accurate population health assessments and benchmarks as well as designing group-specific health interventions. No such federal data collection has ever occurred in the same magnitude up to date.

Despite these important emerging advances in data disaggregation (Panapasa et al., 2011; CDC, 2017; Wu & Bakos, 2017), systemic lack of data disaggregation continues to negatively affect the health of the AANHPI communities due to a lack of access to data about our own communities. This is in part because U.S. federal and state governments and other organizations continue to use the "Asian Pacific Islander" category despite the official changes from the U.S. Office of Management and Budget. The serious implications of lack of data disaggregation became more apparent in the current and ongoing COVID-19 pandemic contexts. In most states, Asian Americans and Pacific Islanders are aggregated within the "Asian Pacific Islander" category; it greatly masks the stark differences between Asian Americans and Pacific Islanders. Without adjusting for population characteristics differences, it is estimated that nearly one in 1,670 Asian Americans (or 59.9 deaths per 100,000) and one in 895 Pacific Islanders (or 112.0 deaths per 100,000) have died due to COVID-19 (APM, 2020). These incident rates are substantially different from White Americans (one in 1,030 or 97.2 deaths per 100,000) where Asian Americans appear significantly better off whereas Pacific Islanders appear significantly worse off (APM, 2020). In fact, after adjusting for age differences in populations, Pacific Islanders have the worst rates of COVID-19 deaths compared to any other racial/ethnic groups, where Pacific Islanders are 2.5 times more likely to die from COVID-19 compared to White Americans (Kaholokula et al., 2020; APM, 2020; Samoa et al., 2020).

The need for more nuanced second-level data disaggregation is also demonstrated when looking at varying Asian American experiences during the pandemic. The aggregated numbers for Asian Americans are greatly misleading, as they do not show the excessive deaths from COVID-19. Put differently, Asian Americans' mortality advantage prior to the pandemic (i.e., Asian Americans die at older age given the same cause which translates to longer life expectancy) (Acciai et al., 2015) contributed to the invisibility of COVID-19 deaths. In fact, calculating the attributable mortality rates of COVID-19 (i.e., proportion of COVID-19 deaths out of the total number of deaths from all causes including COVID-19) reveals that Asian Americans have been disproportionally affected by COVID-19 as well (Chu et al., 2021). Nearly 13.8% of Asian Americans' deaths can be attributable to COVID-19, a rate substantially higher than that of the U.S. total population (9.2%), and the third highest proportion after Latinx (21.3%) and Black Americans (14.1%). The attributable mortality for Native Hawaiians or Other Pacific Islander was 12.7% (Chu et al., 2021).

Additional significant differences in experiences with COVID-19 are found within the "Asian American" and the "Pacific Islander" panethnic categories. For example, Filipinx nurses account for nearly 30% of all COVID-19 deaths among registered nurses despite only making up about 4% of the total U.S. nurse population (Thomas, 2020). Similarly, although Native Hawaiian and Pacific Islanders are disproportionally affected by COVID-19, overall, emerging numbers show substantial variations among Pacific Islanders as well (McElfish, 2021). Marshallese people are especially hit hard in particular – in northwest Arkansas, the Marshallese population makes up only 1.5% and 3.0% of Benton and Washington counties, yet they accounted for more than 19% of all COVID-19 cases in both counties (Center et al., 2020). In short, the current health emergencies brought by the pandemic have re-affirmed the critical importance of data aggregation for the AANHPI population at both levels.

Data Disaggregation in Action: A Three-Step Example of How Data Disaggregation Matters Using Population Data

In this section, we use the 2014–2015 U.S. natality file from the National Center for Health Statistics (NCHS) of the CDC to show how data disaggregation can unmask the hidden and meaningful differences between and within Asian Americans and Pacific Islanders with actual numbers (National Center for Health Statistics, 2015). Natality data is the population data (as opposed to the survey sampled data), containing all U.S. live birth information from the birth certificates from 50 states, District of Columbia, and U.S. territories. Use of this unique population data allows for assessing the health needs of AANHPI populations that are often not possible with survey data (Yellow Horse & Patterson, 2022).

We focused on two sexually transmitted infections as the outcomes of interest: chlamydia and hepatitis B. The first outcome, chlamydia, is the most common bacterial sexually transmitted infection, in general and during pregnancy (Tiller, 2002). Hepatitis B is the second most common sexually transmitted infection during pregnancy (more prevalent than gonorrhea, syphilis, hepatitis C, and other sexually transmitted infections), but is often an overlooked aspect of pregnant women's experiences with sexually transmitted infections (Borgia et al., 2012; Jonas, 2009). This is in part because hepatitis B infects an individual's liver – rather than genitalia – even though it can be primarily transmitted through sexual activities and there is no cure for hepatitis B unlike chlamydia (Jonas, 2009). Despite the differences in the affected areas and permanence between chlamydia and hepatitis B, both sexually transmitted infections may substantially impact the overall health of mothers and their babies, and both are important aspects of women's sexual and reproductive health during pregnancy (Borgia et al., 2012; Noah, 2018). We also selected these two outcomes as the illustrative examples because AANHPI women's rates of contracting these two sexually transmitted infections are polarized; AANHPI women have the lowest rate of contracting chlamydia and the highest rate of contracting hepatitis B during pregnancy (Noah, 2018).

Step 1. Prevalence of Race/Ethnic Group-Specific Births with Chlamydia and Hepatitis B without Any Data Disaggregation (Using the "AANHPI" Category)

Table 2.1 and Figure 2.1 show the percentage of live births with chlamydia and hepatitis B for multiple race/ethnic groups. In the two-year period of 2014–2015, 7,706,870 births occurred in the United States. Of those births, about 1.83% and 0.22% of the births occurred with the presence of chlamydia and hepatitis B, respectively. AANHPI pregnant women had the smallest percentage of births with chlamydia, which presented in about 0.56% of all births for AANHPI pregnant women. On the other hand, AANHPI pregnant women had the largest percentage of births with hepatitis B, which presented in about 1.68% of all births for AANHPI pregnant women – about 7.3 times higher rate than the overall U.S. population rate (all mothers who have given live births during the two-year period).

Table 2.1 Percent of Race/Ethnic Group-Specific Births with Chlamydia and Hepatitis B in the U.S.

	# Births	*Chlamydia*	*Hepatitis B*
Non-Hispanic White	4,103,761	1.17%	0.08%
Non-Hispanic Black	1,098,154	4.38%	0.36%
Hispanic	1,799,306	1.92%	0.08%
AANHPI	**488,178**	**0.56%**	**1.68%**
Asian Americans	**470,220**	**0.44%**	**1.70%**
Pacific Islanders	**17,958**	**3.66%**	**1.26%**
AIAN	64,616	4.76%	0.09%
Multiracial	152,855	3.01%	0.19%
Total U.S. Population	**7,706,870**	**1.83%**	**0.22%**

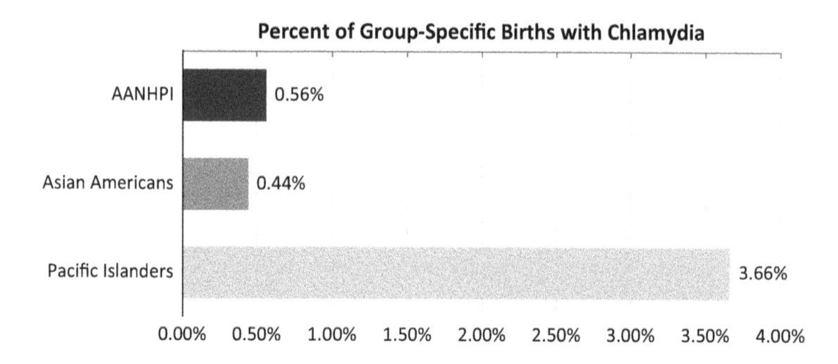

Figure 2.1 First-level Disaggregation of Percent of Group-Specific Births with Chlamydia.

Step 2. Prevalence of Group-Specific Births with Chlamydia and Hepatitis B for Asian American Pregnant Women vs. Pacific Islander Pregnant Women (The first-level data disaggregation)

When the prevalence of group-specific births with chlamydia and hepatitis B is considered separately for Asian American pregnant women and Pacific Islander women, important differences come to light (see Table 2.1, Rows 4–5). The group difference between Asian American pregnant women and Pacific Islander pregnant women is especially stark for chlamydia. When we used the first-level data disaggregation, the numbers show that the percentage of births with chlamydia (see Figure 2.1) for Asian American pregnant women was 0.44%, while the percentage of births with chlamydia for Pacific Islander pregnant women was nearly 3.66% – substantially higher than the percentage when the AANHPI category was used (0.56% for AANHPI). On the other hand, the numbers for births with hepatitis B (see Figure 2.2) show that Asian American

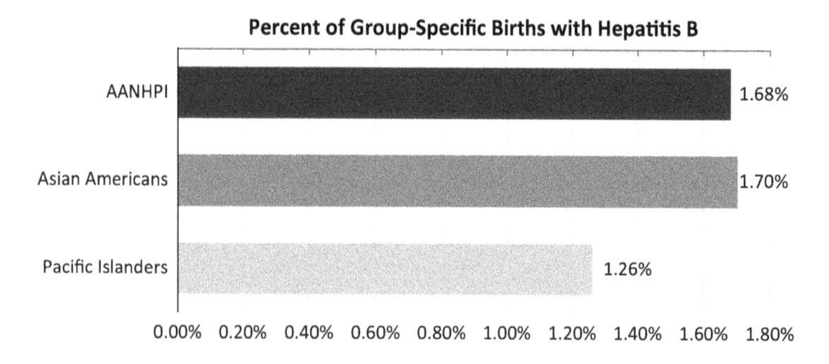

Figure 2.2 First-level Disaggregation of Percent of Group-Specific Births with Hepatitis B.

pregnant women have a higher percentage of births with hepatitis B (1.70%) compared to Pacific Islander pregnant women (1.26%).

Step 3. Prevalence of Group-Specific Births with Chlamydia and Hepatitis B within AANHPI Pregnant Women by Country of Origin (The second-level data disaggregation)

Similar to what we observed in Step 2, when the prevalence of group-specific births with chlamydia and hepatitis B is considered separately for AANHPI pregnant women by their countries of origin, significant differences emerge (see Table 2.2). For example, when we compared the percentages of births with hepatitis B among Asian American pregnant women, Chinese American pregnant women reported the largest percentage (3.47%) and Japanese American pregnant women reported the smallest percentage (0.14%). The numbers for both groups substantially differed from the group mean of 1.70% for all Asian American pregnant women. When we compared the percentages of births with hepatitis B among Pacific Islander pregnant women, important distinctions emerged among Hawaiian (0.18%), Guamanian (0.11%), Sāmoan (0.43%), and "Other Pacific Islanders" (1.99%). The numbers show that the relatively largest size of "Other Pacific Islanders" within the Pacific Islander category (making up about 57.2% of all births among Pacific Islander pregnant women) drives up the group mean to 1.26% – which does not reflect the experiences of any specific group among Pacific Islander pregnant women.

Table 2.2 Percent of Ethnic Group-Specific Births with Chlamydia and Hepatitis B within "AANHPI" Pregnant Women by Country of Origin

	# Births	*Chlamydia*	*Hepatitis B*
AANHPI	**488,178**	**0.56%**	**1.68%**
Asian Americans	***470,220***	***0.44%***	***1.70%***
Asian Indian	127,485	0.13%	0.27%
Chinese	114,020	0.36%	3.47%
Filipino	61,023	0.83%	0.71%
Japanese	13,845	0.32%	0.14%
Korean	28,700	0.26%	1.21%
Vietnamese	40,252	0.59%	3.44%
Other Asian	84,895	0.75%	1.78%
Pacific Islanders	***17,958***	***3.66%***	***1.26%***
Hawaiian	1701	1.41%	0.18%
Guamanian	1819	2.75%	0.11%
Sāmoan	4,172	3.64%	0.43%
Other Islanders	10,266	4.20%	1.99%
Total U.S. Population	**7,706,870**	**1.83%**	**0.22%**

Data Disaggregation in Action: AANHPI Women's Health in Arizona Using Survey Data

In addition to illustrating how two-level data disaggregation can be important for understanding AANHPI women's health, we share the descriptive characteristics from survey data we have collected in the Arizona Asian American and Pacific Islander Women's Health Project.

Table 2.3 shows the descriptive characteristics of women who participated in the project. The first column shows the descriptive characteristics of all women who would be grouped together using the umbrella "AAPI" category. The second column and third column show the descriptive characteristics for Asian American women and Pacific Islander women, respectively. Both Asian American women and Pacific Islander women were similar in age on average (48.6 years old for Asian American women and 49.0 years old for Pacific Islander women) and lived almost two decades in Arizona at the time of the survey. However, when we begin to look at sociodemographic and family characteristics with the first-level data disaggregation, Asian American women and Pacific Islander women have substantially different characteristics. For example, on average, the majority of the women (70.8%) appear to be married or cohabitating with a partner when all "AAPI" women were grouped together. However, when we use the first-level data disaggregation, only about one-third of Asian American women (36.4%) were married or cohabitating compared to all Pacific Islander women (100%). This shows that without data disaggregation, the average

Table 2.3 Descriptive Information of Participants in Focus Group Interviews

	Total/Average (AAPI)	*Asian Americans*	*Pacific Islanders*
Number (n)	24	11	13
Age	48.8	48.6	49.0
Foreign-born	75.0%	63.6%	84.6%
Years in Arizona	18.1	19.8	17.2
College education and beyond	29.2%	45.5%	15.4%
Employment status (Employed)	54.2%	81.8%	30.8%
Marital status (Married and cohabitation)	70.8%	36.4%	100.0%
Number of children	2.91	1.36	4.00
Good self-rated health	91.7%	90.9%	92.3%
Currently using contraception	20.8%	27.3%	15.4%

number for all "AAPI" women does not reflect the realities of either Asian American women or Pacific Islander women. Similarly, while Asian American women have 1.36 children on average, Pacific Islander women have 4.0 children on average.

An across-group difference between Asian American women and Pacific Islander women is also apparent when we look at the percentage of women currently using contraception. Although the average ages and the percentages of women who self-rated their health as good are similar for Asian American women and Pacific Islander women, more than one in four Asian American women shared that they are currently using contraception (27.3%), whereas less than one in six Pacific Islander women are currently using contraception (15.4%).

Given the small sample size of women in the Arizona Asian American and Pacific Islander Women's Health Project, it is difficult to do the second-level data disaggregation to look at ethnic group differences within Asian American women and within Pacific Islander women. As mentioned earlier, this is a common shortcoming with most survey data, even including nationally representative surveys; it demonstrates the need for data to expand to include narrative perspectives. A few examples of voices from the focus groups around the ideas about pregnancy and contraception hint at how the meanings and communications around sexual and reproductive health can differ meaningfully across groups. For example, one of our participants (a first-generation Asian American woman) shared about the lack of communication about sexual and reproductive health in her family:

> I think in terms of sex education, or sexual health – at home it was never talked about. [...] It was kind of this unspoken thing. And then in college when I said I had a boyfriend my mom said something like why do you have to have a boyfriend? So that's how sexuality was not talked about, and birth control was not talked about it was not addressed at all.

Another participant shared a contrasting experience around sexual and reproductive health in her family:

> Because they are having, they are just having their period. Then mom explains to them, "Now you have your period and you are a woman. So you have to take care of yourself because now it's open anytime you can be pregnant you know."

Moving Forward with Data Disaggregation or Not? Intersectionality and More Complexities

The three-step example of data disaggregation using the natality population data and the example of data disaggregation using the Arizona Asian American and Pacific Islander Women's Health Project survey data show that we miss out on important nuances and group differences within AANHPI pregnant women without data disaggregation. Not only do Asian American pregnant women and Pacific Islander pregnant women differ on birth outcomes as two panethnic groups (shown by the results from the first-level data disaggregation), but there were also substantial and meaningful differences within those two categories by women's countries of origin (shown by the results from the second-level data disaggregation).

In addition to important differences at the individual level, important differences of broader social contexts also exist. For example, the concentration of Asian Americans and Pacific Islanders in certain regions and metropolitan areas is another factor that also must be taken into account when discussing public health. Metropolitan areas with higher proportions of AANHPI residents will be more likely to pay attention to AANHPI health concerns than those areas with lower representation. AANHPIs are less likely to live in rural areas. It would not be surprising for certain health practitioners, depending on where they were trained and where they grew up, to lack familiarity with the diversity of AANHPIs culturally and in relation to health issues. The lack of attention to and knowledge about AANHPI health specifically has repercussions for all AANHPIs. Questions of citizenship among AANHPI women matter particularly in relation to access to federal programs like Medicaid and Medicare.

Debating the strengths and limitations of data aggregation versus data disaggregation raises an important question: How do we simultaneously advocate for data aggregation for collective "strength in numbers" for political representation while demanding data, which allow our diverse AANHPI communities to assess and address our own with-in group issues? On a related note, recognizing our communities' diversity also requires us to consider how we think about the intersectional struggles within and across groups.

Notes

1 These numbers from the 1960 U.S. Census do not mean that there were no other Asian American or Pacific Islander groups. Only three Asian subgroups and no Pacific Islander groups being represented in the Census is due to how certain groups were systemically erased from data representation based on which categories were available in data collection (Sasa & Yellow Horse, 2022). For example, the first Korean immigrants to the United States (i.e., Hawaii) were in 1903 (Patterson, 1994).

2 We caution the interpretation of the "household income" for AANHPI families as AANHPI individuals are more likely to reside in multi-generational households and have multiple adults contributing to the overall household income. For example, in 2019, nearly 87.3 percent of Asian Americans and 90.5 percent of Pacific Islanders reported living in some type of family households (i.e., not living alone or living in nonfamily households) – compared to 87.3 percent for non-Hispanic/Latinx White individuals. It is estimated that about 26 percent of Asian Americans reside in multigenerational households, which is substantially higher than the U.S. overall rate (19 percent) (López, Ruiz, & Patten, 2017). In particular, non-married AANHPI adults are more likely to reside in the same households with their parents; thus, the value of "household income" for AANHPI households is likely inflated due to multiple adults contributing income to the household.

3 There are two mechanisms for population growth: immigration (incoming of individuals from other countries) and natural growth (new individuals in a population from childbirth). Although the Hispanic/Latinx community also has a large proportion of foreign-born members, the population growth of Hispanic/Latinx is driven by natural growth (i.e., high fertility rate) (Lopez et al., 2017).

4 Pacific Islanders are conflated with other "numerically small non-Hispanic race" (i.e., American Indian and Alaskan Native populations) under the umbrella of "Indigenous" population.

5 Distrust is "a measure of how much the truster believes that the trustee will actively work against them in a given situation" (Marsh & Dibben 2005: p. 20). It is based on reliable information and experiences, and not just a general sense of unease (i.e., mistrust).

References

Acciai, F., Noah, A. J., & Firebaugh, G. (2015). Pinpointing the sources of the Asian mortality advantage in the USA. *Journal of Epidemiology Community Health*, *69*(10), 1006–1011. 10.1136/jech-2015-205623

APM Research Lab (APM)., (2020). The color of coronavirus: Covid-19 deaths by race and ethnicity in the US. *APM Research Lab.*

Arfken, M. (2013). Social justice and the politics of recognition. *American Psychologist*, *68*(6), 475–480. https://psycnet.apa.org/doi/10.1037/a0033596

Bitton, A., Zaslavsky, A. M., & Ayanian, J. Z. (2010). Health risks, chronic diseases, and access to care among US Pacific Islanders. *Journal of General Internal Medicine*, *25*(5), 435–440. 10.1007/s11606-009-1241-0

Borgia, G., Carleo, M. A., Gaeta, G. B., & Gentile, I. (2012). Hepatitis B in pregnancy. *World Journal of Gastroenterology*, *18*(34), 4677. doi:10.3748/wjg.v18.i34.4677

Center, K. E., Da Silva, J., Hernandez, A. L., Vang, K., Martin, D. W., Mazurek, J., … & Campbell, E. M. (2020). Multidisciplinary community-based investigation of a COVID-19 outbreak among Marshallese and Hispanic/Latino communities—Benton and Washington Counties, Arkansas, March–June 2020. *Morbidity and Mortality Weekly Report*, *69*(48), 1807. 10.15585/mmwr.mm6948a2

Center, P. R. (2020). *What Census Calls US*. Retrieved from Washington DC: https://www.pewresearch.org/interactives/what-census-calls-us/

Centers for Disease Control and Prevention (CDC) (2017). Native Hawaiian and Pacific Islander (NHPI) National Health Interview Survey (NHIS). Retrieved from https://www.cdc.gov/nchs/nhis/nhpi.html

Chu, J. N., Tsoh, J. Y., Ong, E., & Ponce, N. A. (2021). The hidden colors of coronavirus: The burden of attributable COVID-19 deaths. *Journal of General Internal Medicine*, 1–3. 10.1007/s11606-020-06497-4

Cohn, D. (2015). *Future immigration will change the face of America by 2065*. Retrieved from Washington DC: https://www.pewresearch.org/fact-tank/2015/10/05/future-immigration-will-change-the-face-of-america-by-2065/

Cokley, K., & Awad, G. H. (2013). In defense of quantitative methods: Using the "master's tools" to promote social justice. *Journal for Social Action in Counseling & Psychology*, *5*(2), 26–41. 10.33043/JSACP.5.2.26-41

Espiritu, Y. L. (1993). *Asian American panethnicity: Bridging institutions and identities*. Philadelphia, PA: Temple University Press.

Hooker, K., Phibbs, S., Irvin, V. L., Mendez-Luck, C. A., Doan, L. N., Li, T., … & Choun, S. (2019). Depression among older adults in the United States by disaggregated race and ethnicity. *The Gerontologist*, *59*(5), 886–891. 10.1093/geront/gny159

Humes, K., & Hogan, H. (2009). Measurement of race and ethnicity in a changing, multicultural America. *Race and Social Problems*, *1*(3), 111–115. 10.1007/s12552-009-9011-5

Jonas, M. M. (2009). Hepatitis B and pregnancy: An underestimated issue. *Liver international*, *29*, 133–139. 10.1111/j.1478-3231.2008.01933.x

Kaholokula, J. K., Okamoto, S. K., & Yee, B. W. (2019). Special issue introduction: Advancing Native Hawaiian and other Pacific Islander health. *Asian American Journal of Psychology*, *10*(3), 197–205. 10.1037/aap0000167

Kaholokula, J. K., Samoa, R. A., Miyamoto, R. E., Palafox, N., & Daniels, S.-A. (2020). COVID-19 special column: COVID-19 hits native Hawaiian and Pacific Islander communities the hardest. *Hawai'i Journal of Health & Social Welfare*, *79*(5), 144.

Kindig, D. A., Asada, Y., & Booske, B. (2008). A population health framework for setting national and state health goals. *Jama*, *299*(17), 2081–2083. doi:10.1001/jama.299.17.2081

Kochhar, R., & Cilluffo, A. (2018). Income inequality in the US is rising most rapidly among Asians. *Pew Research Center*.

Lee, E. (2015). *The making of Asian America: A history*. New York, NY: Simon and Schuster.

Lee, E. (2019). *America for Americans: A history of xenophobia in the United States*. New York, NY: Basic Books.

Locke, J. T. (2009). Climate change-induced migration in the Pacific Region: Sudden crisis and long-term developments. *Geographical Journal*, *175*(3), 171–180. 10.1111/j.1475-4959.2008.00317.x

López, G., Ruiz, N. G., & Patten, E. (2017). *Key facts about Asian Americans, a diverse and growing population*. Retrieved from Washington DC: https://www.pewresearch.org/fact-tank/2017/09/08/key-facts-about-asian-americans/

Marsh, S., & Dibben, M. R. (2005). *Trust, untrust, distrust and mistrust–An exploration of the dark (er) side*. Paper presented at the International Conference on Trust Management.

Mau, M. K., Sinclair, K., Saito, E. P., Baumhofer, K. N., & Kaholokula, J. K. (2009). Cardiometabolic health disparities in native Hawaiians and other Pacific Islanders. *Epidemiologic Reviews*, *31*(1), 113–129. 10.1093/ajerev/mxp004

Mays, V. M., Ponce, N. A., Washington, D. L., & Cochran, S. D. (2003). Classification of race and ethnicity: Implications for public health. *Annual Review of Public Health*, *24*(1), 83–110. 10.1146/annurev.publhealth.24.100901.140927

McElfish, P. A. (2021). COVID-19 disparities among Marshallese Pacific Islanders. *Preventing Chronic Disease*, *18*, E02. 10.5888/pcd18.200407

McGeeney, K., Kriz, B., Mullenax, S., Kail, L., Walejko, G., Vines, M., … & García, Y. (2019). *2020 census barriers, attitudes, and motivators study survey report*. Retrieved from Suitland, MD: https://www.census.gov/programs-surveys/decennial-census/2020-census/planning-management/final-analysis/2020-report-cbams-study-survey.html

National Center for Health Statistics (2015). *Natality public-use data file and documentation*. National Center for Health Statistics.

Nguyen, B.-M. D., Nguyen, M. H., & Nguyen, T.-L. K. (2013). Advancing the Asian American and Pacific Islander data quality campaign: Data disaggregation practice and policy. *Asian American Policy Review*, *24*, 55.

Noah, A. J. (2018). Heterogeneity of Hepatitis B Infection Among Pregnant Asian American and Pacific Islander Women. *American journal of preventive medicine*, *55*(2), 213–221. 10.1016/j.amepre.2018.03.021

Nobles, M. (2000). *Shades of citizenship: Race and the census in modern politics*. Stanford University Press.

Okamoto, D. G. (2003). Toward a theory of panethnicity: Explaining Asian American collective action. *American Sociological Review*, *68*(6), 811–842. 10.2307/1519747

Okamoto, D. G. (2014). *Redefining race: Asian American panethnicity and shifting ethnic boundaries*. Russell Sage Foundation.

Omi, M., & Winant, H. (1994). *Racial formation in the United States: From the 1960s to the 1990s*. Routledge.

Panapasa, S., Crabbe, K., & Kaholokula, J. K. (2011). Efficacy of federal data: Revised office of management and budget standard for native Hawaiian and other Pacific Islanders examined. *AAPI Nexus: Policy, Practice and Community*, *9*(1–2), 212–220. doi:10.17953/appc.9.1-2.cp21x04488016643

Patterson, W. (1994). *The Korean Frontier in America: Immigration to Hawaii, 1896–1910*. Honolulu, HI: University of Hawaii Press.

Rowse, T. (2012). *Rethinking social justice: From'peoples' to 'populations'*. Aboriginal Studies Press.

Samoa, R., Kaholokula, J. K., Penaia, C., Tupai-Firestone, R., Fa'amoe-Timoteo, E., Laelan, M., & Aitaoto, N. (2020). COVID-19 and the state of health of Pacific Islanders in the United States. *AAPI Nexus*, *17*(1&2), 1–17. https://escholarship.org/uc/item/1q00k9c4

Sasa, S. M., & Yellow Horse, A. J. (2022). Just data representation for Native Hawaiians and Pacific Islanders: A critical review of systemic Indigenous erasure in census and recommendations for psychologists. *American journal of community psychology*, *69*(3–4), 343–354. 10.1002/ajcp.12569

Seltzer, W., & Anderson, M. (2007). *Census confidentiality under the second war powers act (1942–1947)*. Paper presented at the Population Association of America annual meeting, New York, NY.

Spickard, P., Rondilla, J. L., & Wright, D. H. (2002). *Pacific diaspora: Island peoples in the United States and across the Pacific*. University of Hawaii Press.

Srinivasan, S., & Guillermo, T. (2000). Toward improved health: disaggregating Asian American and Native Hawaiian/Pacific Islander data. *American journal of public health*, *90*(11), 1731–1734. 10.2105%2Fajph.90.11.1731

Taualii, M., Quenga, J., Samoa, R., Samanani, S., & Dover, D. (2011). Liberating data: Accessing Native Hawaiian and Other Pacific Islander data from national data sets. *AAPI Nexus: Policy, Practice and Community*, *9*(1–2), 249–255.

Teranishi, R. T., Nguyen, B. M. D., & Alcantar, C. M. (2014). The Asian American and Pacific Islander data disaggregation movement: The convergence of community activism and policy reform. *Asian American Policy Review*, *25*, 26–36.

Thomas, K. (2020). COVID exacts high toll among Filipino nurses — Recent data provide context for this risk. *MedPage Today*. Retrieved from https://www.medpagetoday.com/nursing/nursing/88812

Tiller, C. M. (2002). Chlamydia during pregnancy: Implications and impact on perinatal and neonatal outcomes. *Journal of Obstetric, Gynecologic, & Neonatal Nursing*, *31*(1), 93–98. 10.1111/j.1552-6909.2002.tb00027.x

Tiongson Jr, A. T. (2019). Asian American studies, comparative racialization, and settler colonial critique. *Journal of Asian American Studies*, *22*(3), 419–443. 10.1353/jaas.2019.0030

Tran, V. C., Lee, J., Khachikian, O., & Lee, J. (2018). Hyper-selectivity, racial mobility, and the remaking of race. *RSF: The Russell Sage Foundation Journal of the Social Sciences*, *4*(5), 188–209. 10.7758/RSF.2018.4.5.09

U.S. Office of Management and Budget (OMB), (1997). *Race and Ethnic Standards for Federal Statistics and Administrative Reporting*. Retrieved from Washington, DC: https://www.census.gov/srd/papers/pdf/sm97-08.pdf

U.S. Census Bureau, (1960). *1960 Decennial Census*; generated by Aggie J. Yellow Horse; using American Factfinder; http://factfinder2.census.gov

U.S. Census Bureau, (2019). *2015–2019 American Community Survey 5-Year Estimates*; generated by Aggie J. Yellow Horse; using American Factfinder; http://factfinder2.census.gov

U.S. Census Bureau, (2020). Importance of the Data. Retrieved from https://2020census.gov/en/census-data.html

Wong, M. M., Klingle, R. S., & Price, R. K. (2004). Alcohol, tobacco, and other drug use among Asian American and Pacific Islander adolescents in California and Hawaii. *Addictive behaviors*, *29*(1), 127–141. 10.1016/S0306-4603(03)00079-0

Wu, S., & Bakos, A. (2017). The native Hawaiian and Pacific Islander National Health Interview Survey: Data collection in small populations. *Public Health Reports*, *132*(6), 606–608. 10.1177/0033354917729181

Yellow Horse, A. J., & Patterson, S. E. (2022). Greater inclusion of Asian Americans in aging research on family caregiving for better understanding of racial health inequities. *The Gerontologist*, *62*(5), 704–710. 10.1093/geront/gnab156

Young, M. C., Gerber, M. W., Ash, T., Horan, C. M., & Taveras, E. M. (2018). Neighborhood social cohesion and sleep outcomes in the Native Hawaiian and Pacific Islander National Health Interview Survey. *Sleep*, *41*(9), zsy097. 10.1093/sleep/zsy097

Zhou, M., & Lee, J. (2017). Hyper-selectivity and the remaking of culture: Understanding the Asian American achievement paradox. *Asian American Journal of Psychology*, *8*(1), 7–15. https://psycnet.apa.org/doi/10.1037/aap0000069

Zia, H. (2000). *Asian American dreams: The emergence of an American people*. Farrar, Straus, & Giroux.

3 Self Representation: AANHPI Storytelling About Sexual and Reproductive Health

> But as far as sharing to the next generation it's not always the same, right? So behind doors – we'll talk about sexual health and like things like that. But talk about it in public? You know it's a scary-like feeling. But we need to have conversations, it's a healthy conversation.
>
> *-Kasey, Focus group participant*

The opening quote of this section captures one of the key reasons we chose to focus on sexual and reproductive health in this project: "We need to have conversations, it's a healthy conversation." Whereas Chapter 2 provided an overview of data related to Asian American, Native Hawaiian and Pacific Islander (AANHPI) women's health, this chapter provides a personal perspective into ways that AANHPI women think and learn about sexual and reproductive health. Many AANHPI women learn *not* to have these conversations. We wanted to better understand where and how these lessons about sexual and reproductive health were learned and to what extent they were connected to areas of diversity such as culture, race, gender, religion, and immigrant background. In our focus groups, we centered on storytelling as a method for gathering information on topics that many women, especially AANHPI women, rarely speak about with others. We found that our participants were willing to share everyday stories of sexual health and health care, memories of learning about reproductive health and ways that these stories changed how they make choices in their own lives, particularly in communication with their children. In general, these stories were often told with humor and self-reflection. (See Appendix A for the initial script we used in our focus groups.)

The stories generated in our focus groups contrasted with many of the traumatic stories overrepresented in narratives about the sexuality of women of color and many of the "model minority" stories as represented by aggregated data of AANHPI. Many moments in our focus groups were joyful and funny and suggested ways of building new connections

DOI: 10.4324/9781003449867-4

for the participants. The conversations and stories also helped us to consider more creative ways to structure further outreach and education, as we explore in the next chapter.

As we thought about how to approach and encourage Asian American and Pacific Islander women to speak about their own experiences with sexual and reproductive health, we (the authors) recalled our own experiences. How and why would we be willing to discuss these topics with researchers? How did we initially learn about sexual and reproductive health? A narrative and storytelling mechanism seemed a good method, providing a means of tapping into micro and macro ways of learning. We tell stories to ourselves about our past, present, and future and as a way of sharing cultural knowledge from generation to generation. Stories hold a lot of weight: memories of family traditions, successes and failures, favorite foods and immigration are all preserved and shared from generation to generation through stories. Health stories are sometimes hidden within these, revealed in a description of a tradition related to a certain stage of life (e.g., puberty) or a discussion of the healing properties of a food. But these stories, and the underlying cultural practices and knowledge, are rarely discussed in relation to health. For example, one of our focus group participants recalled how all the foods she was used to eating suddenly became off-limits after surgery, like turmeric. She said, "I went to class on what things I can eat, but the Asian part of the food was never discussed."

Our method of seeking stories within focus groups sought to highlight some of the complex ways these Asian Americans and Pacific Islander women, some who immigrated as children, some who immigrated as adults, some who are second or third generation, thought about their health generally and sexual and reproductive health in particular. We focused on first memories related to sexual and reproductive health and on "period stories" as one event related to sexual and reproductive health that often function as a "flashbulb memory" – an autobiographical memory that is of special importance and carries specific details about meaning, time and place (Brown & Kulik, 1977). For example, one of the authors remembers never seeing any products related to menstruation present in her house until she began her own period, at which point she could recall specific details about her mom taking her into a darkened bedroom and sitting on her parents' bed with its white chintz bedspread and watching her mom wordlessly pull a package with sanitary pads and a sanitary belt out of the middle drawer from the dresser. Similarly, many of our participants could recall specific details around this event. Drawing out these memories also sometimes revealed details related to family traditions, cultural practices and beliefs, and ways of talking about sex. Woven in with these specific stories were details about lessons learned in relation to sexuality and how these were conveyed based on age and gender and how they might have influenced current sexual and reproductive health practices for the participants. One key question we wanted to consider in gathering stories was how do the stories we have learned and the ones we tell ourselves influence the decisions we make about our health?

Okazaki's (2002) review of the literature on how culture influences sexual attitudes of Asian and Asian American women found that AA women tend to be more "conservative" in their attitudes toward sex. She points out that although erotica in many Asian cultures has existed for centuries, talk about sex was restricted to married couples and strict attitudes within some Asian ethnic groups were connected to Christian religious influences. In Okazaki's review, many studies found that Asian American adolescents and college students tended to be more sexually conservative than their peers, with lower levels of sexual knowledge and lower rates of sexual experience. She also found that there was lower engagement with sexual and reproductive health practices (such as breast cancer screening) as adults, which she speculated might be related to the lack of communication, knowledge and experience about sexual and reproductive health in adolescence and early adulthood. As Okazaki (2002) concluded, "there appears to be a pervasive tendency for Asian American girls and women to be more reluctant than White American girls and women to seek care for their sexual and reproductive health" (p. 38).

In their article "Communicating Reproduction" (Hopwood et al., 2015), the authors discuss how knowledge is shared and circulated involved in understanding and discussing reproduction throughout history. They detail how print technology and books allowed knowledge about sex to be shared more widely and the ways in which the language of reproduction came to be shaped by men – how male doctors became the "experts" at the expense of women's individual knowledge. However, they also trace and examine the ways that narratives and storytelling underlie much of the knowledge. Ultimately, expert knowledge is framed and shaped by individual stories: "A repertoire, drawn from biblical or classical sources or rooted in local lore, laboratory procedure, or everyday experience, has inflected what we say and how" (Hopwood et al., 2015, p. 309). This interplay between everyday knowing and expert knowledge continues to shape the understanding of sexual and reproductive health for women. Using personal stories as the starting point for our discussions elevates the everyday knowing and may uncover the cultural and generational narratives that influence how AANHPI women approach their own health. Tracing these stories must also acknowledge not just culture, race, gender and immigration status, but also complex histories of colonization, as the stories and experiences many AANHPI women relate have a direct connection to the ways in which U.S. military and religious institutions affected their families and communities.

Chapter 1 of this book provides a broader historical and social context for interpreting and understanding the stories of AANHPI women – including drawing on the research of feminist disability studies. As Garland-Thomson (2005) explained, "Feminist disability studies not only retrieves overlooked experiences … it strives to rewrite oppressive social scripts" (p. 1567). By supporting and uncovering little-told narratives of AANHPI women's sexual and reproductive experiences, this work can "reimagine" the stereotypes placed upon AANHPI women. As with feminist disability studies, we hope our project "centers on revising cultural narratives" (Garland-Thomson, 2005, p. 1567) around women's AANHPI sexual and reproductive health.

In this chapter, we consider the importance of this storytelling framework for better understanding AANHPI women's health. What stories do AANHPI women tell about sexual and reproductive health and how have their own choices been shaped and changed by these stories? We specifically consider a) why the storytelling method was important to our work, b) how storytelling transformed the focus group into communal space that allowed individuals to address topics they did not typically discuss, c) ways that stories spark generative interpretations for both participants and researchers and d) the role of stories as symbolic "companions" (Frank, 2010) for navigating sexual and reproductive health for AANHPI women. Throughout, we also discuss some of the common themes and elements and the strengths and weaknesses of this work. Finally, we speculate on the role of humor in health stories and how this may support further community conversations around issues of sexual and reproductive health.

Navigating History and Tradition

Storytelling invokes history and tradition, even when done in a focus group setting. Stories are typically considered to include the main character, a problem and some personal lesson learned. Stories will also often involve an element of performance. Warren (2008) highlights storytelling as performance and her emphasis on the importance of the images and emotions evoked for both the teller and audience are especially key in a focus group setting. The ways in which stories are told and others connect to them help audience members – or in our case other focus group participants – to examine the ways their own lives may compare and contrast with the storyteller's experience.

Some scholars distinguish between a narrative and a story (e.g., Bradby, 2017; Wong & Breheny, 2018), with story referring to something more personal and rehearsed (and perhaps fictionalized). Wong and Breheny (2018) argue that narratives reference broader societal structures and meanings, "we make the distinction that a story is the account of events the speaker tells, while a narrative refers to the wider accounts of social life that are drawn upon to tell a story. Consequently, we suggest that people tell stories, and that they use widely available narratives to tell these stories" (p. 246). For our purposes storytelling and narrative are used together, as stories are a means of narrating and giving meaning to our world. Fraser (2004), who sees stories and narratives as working together, discusses the critical ways that they function. In her article on narrative research in social work, she explains "Storytelling is such an important activity because narratives help people to organize their experiences into meaningful episodes that call upon cultural modes of reasoning and representation ..." (Fraser, 2004, p. 180). Asking for a specific story helps individuals to share already framed and organized memories that tap into broader narratives they have about who they are in relation to their past, present and future. Our focus groups utilized stories to allow women to reflect on a moment in their lives and provide meaning to it from both their current perspective and in relation to the context and culture in which they experienced it.

For example, one of our participants, Tess, provided a cultural interpretation to past experiences about the lessons her mother emphasized about sexuality, while also reflecting upon how her upbringing shaped her current political views:

> At one point we used to have braided, pleated hair with oil in our hair. And my mom just could not, did not want me to leave my hair loose. My interpretation is because loose hair maybe is more attractive or is less controlled, I had to fight with her to let me cut my hair, because I wanted to cut my hair. So I felt like sexuality was something that had to be very tightly controlled in girls. Maybe that's also my perspective as a feminist and maybe I'm a feminist because I saw the unequal treatment.

Tess had been discussing how she and her sister had to argue with their mom to be able to shave their legs and that as girls their behaviors and appearance were controlled and monitored in many ways that her brother did not face. Her reflection at the end that she may be interpreting the experience from a feminist viewpoint and simultaneously that her viewpoint may have resulted from her strict upbringing, illustrates the ways in which individuals reflect on the interplay between past and present as they narrate.

Another participant, Anna, explained how she was intent on doing things differently than her mom with her daughters with respect to discussing sex:

> I have four girls, and so when I had my girls, I taught them at a very young age about it. I taught them everything so that they don't run

> into those issues. So again, I don't know if that's a cultural thing or it's because my mom's mom passed at a young age. She (my mom) was young and she really didn't know how to, you know, talk about it. [When I started my period] I was screaming, she ran into the bathroom, she thought that I hurt myself really bad, and I was like hilarious hysterical and I was just screaming and crying. She says, that's okay. So every one of my daughters, I make a big celebration, we go out to lunch, I give her a gift full of pads, you know, I turn it into a *positive* rather than something scary.

Because sexual health is often very private, especially in Asian American families (e.g., Okazaki, 2002), the focus group also became a means of creating a space where stories could "breathe" (Frank, 2010) and participants could see that others shared similar experiences. In their book *Performing Health and Wellbeing*, Baxter and Low (2017) discuss ways that interactive performance allows for exploration of difficult health topics, including sexual health. In a chapter about work with South African students, Low (2017) specifically considers ways that performance can allow spaces to be more open and provide a chance to de-stigmatize conversations regarding sex. Low is discussing a theater space, but our story-based focus groups may serve the same purpose, "It is having that space in which people can individually make sense of the experience that is most resonant" (Low, 2017, p. 153). Beyond the space for this work, the focus group allowed the participants to authenticate their experiences and gain appreciation for those experiences. The building of relationships through authentic storytelling was key. As Low argues, "In order to start conversations around sex and relationships, we need to provide avenues for intimate moments of recognition" (Low, 2017, p. 154).

In the focus groups, the moments of intimate recognition were those that allowed for reassurance, laughter and support. Women would say "yes, yes," nod their heads or add their own insights about a cultural practice that related to sexual and reproductive health. Women offered advice, filled in missing vocabulary ("You know, you know when you're like stop, so like what happens when you stop your pee, you know like that feeling, you're clenching. And so you can even do that just sitting here. Clench your muscles." – "kegels!") and even asked us (the researchers) if we "wanted all this" as they laughed about what they were discussing.

In one focus group, the conversation turned to orgasms and a participant began to wonder aloud whether an aunt who had 10 children had ever had an orgasm. Another participant said she asked her aunt about having sex and told this story:

> One day I was curious at the age of 40 – something [laughter]. I asked my aunt, "So how did you guys have, have sex?" And you know, the old lady said, we just go like this [leans back, waves arms and legs in the air; everyone laughs] so that's why they have 14, 15 kids. Because my aunt told me she just went like ["spread legs" laughter]. That really told me that my mom didn't know what orgasm was, right? Because when my aunt told me she just went like this, and when that husband is done it's done.

One side comment following this story was, "All about the men." This story served as proof to the other women that if all the aunt was doing was lying on her back, it was unlikely she experienced orgasm. The experience was authenticated and appreciated by the other participants, and it reinforced what they also had learned about sex.

The importance of telling the stories in a group is echoed by the work of Parks (2023) who used storytelling in her work on preservice teachers. Parks found storytelling circles generated reflective practice for her participants especially due to the group setting: "In general, narrative research encourages reflection since it requires the storyteller to select an incident, to organize the telling of the incident in a coherent way to illustrate an intended message. The group setting of Story Circles, however, required the narrators to reflect more deeply on their experiences as they negotiated the meaning of their stories with their audience" (p. 67).

The recognition in each other's experiences as women, Asian Americans, Native Hawaiians, and Pacific Islanders, outsiders to U.S. culture and different generations was a key reason that having these conversations in shared spaces, rather than privately, could allow the stories to be reassuring and comforting rather than uncomfortable and strange. By having the participants together, the shared stories and experiences were transformed into humor rather than stigma and the experiences became commonplace rather than out of place.

Creating Liminal Spaces for Community

AANHPI women, especially those from first- or second-generation immigrant families, are used to living in liminal spaces, straddling different cultural practices, languages and expectations with feelings of ambivalence about the various roles that they play in family, community and society. Liminality, a term from anthropology, refers to in-between spaces of transition, sometimes as with physical spaces of transition, sometimes with shifts in time and sometimes in cultural rituals (e.g., Turner, 1998). Liminality has more recently been a concept used in other areas of study, to examine spaces where borders are crossed and power may shift (Carlson et al., 2020).

We knew the focus group needed to take place in an environment outside of the university to allow for easier access to participants. We worked with a local Asian Pacific community health group to use their space for our meeting and this site provided easy parking and was close to a freeway. Andrews and colleagues (2019) discussed how intersectional liminal spaces were critical in gathering data about African Caribbean women's health in the UK. The researchers wanted to provide a space that opened up possibilities for new conversations and utilized talk radio, community groups and hair salons as the intersectional liminal spaces in which to conduct conversations. They describe the importance of the spaces:

> It is in such liminal, *in-between* spaces that exist between public and private where ideas can be formed, reformed, and redefined without the constraints of wider societal conventions. What emerges from the liminal space is not necessarily a definitive answer, but rather an alternative way of understanding social realities where artistic, political, cultural, and social ideas and concepts are in constant flux and contestation. For applied health research, the liminal space gives theoretical grounding for investigations to explore how marginalized people negotiate their health realities. (p. 4)

Andrews and colleagues found that the choice of liminal spaces for data collection was critical to ensuring the African Caribbean women felt comfortable and empowered to discuss health issues. They reflected on this point, "the methodology must allow space for seldom heard knowledges and their creation processes to be acknowledged … the positioning of the research must be able to reflect personal narratives within wider social contexts for understandings that can be used to develop effective health interventions" (p. 3). Our focus groups, held at the site of an AANHPI community health group, provided a similar function in allowing our participants to share their stories and knowledge and delve into discussions away from the "constraints" of typical conventions.

In addition to the physical space, the space formed through storytelling is important in establishing a different context than typical research practices. Using stories to gather data is critical to authenticating the space as one where what is considered appropriate (or not) when discussing health and sex is minimized. Carlson and colleagues (2020) argue for "twisting" liminalities, that "liminalities and liminal spaces call for creative, qualitative methodological problem solving. Maybe new questions, concepts, methods, and interactions with participants could be invented" (p. 1057). Prior to beginning the process, we had not envisioned the ways in which the focus group as a liminal space would seed innovative methods. However, from our conversations and stories in these spaces we were surprised by the ways in which the conversations unfolded, the trust established with the participants and the ways that the focus group became a site of humor. This then sparked experimentation with how results would be presented to the community – working with a performance artist for a larger discussion of the findings (described in chapter 4).

This liminal space also forced us to take into account the role of ambivalence on the part of both researchers and participants. As others (e.g., Frank, 2010) recognize, narratives play many roles – they may or may not be trustworthy, they change over time and are often presented in a way to frame one's self in a certain light. The act of sharing stories as well as the stories themselves contribute to an ambivalence. On the research side, we were probing for stories to better understand AANHPI women's sexual and reproductive health and connections to culture and immigrant experiences, but at the same time we do not want to essentialize AANHPI women or misrepresent their experiences. We knew that discussions of sexual and reproductive health often take place with ambivalence – within families and between parents and children in particular. And from our participants there was sometimes an ambivalence about how much to share and the extent to which they were critical of their past and how this past was reflected in current practices.

One participant, Evie, demonstrated this ambivalence when discussing her desire to share things with her daughters, but how this conflicted with what she was taught by her elders, which was *not* to discuss sexual and reproductive health:

> A mom [has] to share thing[s] they know for their kid … And I think that's the problem. And I was thinking and some time I was angry with my custom because I know custom is really important for people but it's not for the family. We have to share thing[s] for our kid. And just, just me, I was looking at my girl and I says I really wanted to share things … Because they're really young. They won't know anything yet.

Evie discussed responding to her daughters' question about how she became a parent and letting her daughters know it was because their dad and Evie loved each other but that she would explain more when they got older. Evie felt good about this response because as a child her questions were never answered.

As with Evie's response, the focus groups proved to be a generative space for addressing ambivalence, providing an opportunity where women shared in these feelings, transforming the liminal space into one of shared understanding and recognition and mutual dialog between participants and researchers. We especially appreciated the focus groups as an opportunity to reflect on what meaning our stories carry in our lives.

Frank (2010) explains, "research is one occasion for enacting meaning [...] an ongoing dialogue between participants' meaning; the meanings that researchers attribute to their words, their actions, their lives, and their stories; and how participants change in response to researchers' responses" (p. 99).

Interpretations and Connections

Wong and Breheny (2018) provide a detailed model for analyzing narratives in health psychology, where they take into account different levels in which a story may operate: personal, interpersonal, positional and ideological. The personal level is the story told for the individual, providing meaning for the individual. The interpersonal acknowledges that the story is told to an audience and that the teller may shape their story for the audience, with the audience responding or encouraging further elements of the story or with the teller trying to engage or entertain the audience. The positional and ideological levels are the ways that a story functions in relation to broader societal practices. For example, the narrator/storyteller may tell their story from their position as a child and parent and ideologically their story may carry commentary on the treatment of women in society. Wong and Breheny's framework provides a helpful way of considering how a personal story may hold meaning both for the individual and the group, and how these levels shape understandings of health.

Participants in our study spoke both to themselves and to other group members as they shared information, and this provided alternative ways of thinking about health for everyone in the group. In one exchange, the participants were discussing weight and body size.

Cara: So the weight is an issue. People always back home, "Don't gain weight! Don't gain weight!" I was always told. They don't think like Americans – you know, people don't judge you the way you look here (some disagree saying they do judge people here). But not like in Japan! It's horrible.

Researcher: Is that something your family said too?

Cara: Oh yeah, my dad in particular. He said if you're fat you can't get married. (laughter) That mentality – so old school.

Paula: Back home when you gain weight, we call it healthy. And when you're really skinny, there's something wrong with you, you need to eat more. So we look the opposite way of people gaining weight, we say, "They're really healthy."

Didi: It's the same in the Philippines I remember that. They say oh you know you're so skinny you must come from a poor family you don't have any food to eat. But when you're healthy they think oh, you must be a millionaire.

Paula: Back home, we never worry about our weight, it's like small medium large is always the same in our eyes.

The back and forth of this conversation provided an opportunity for comparison of values, oppressive judgements about body size and alternative meanings and interpretations as well as support in resisting the negative messages learned about eating and weight.

The use of stories as a means of understanding requires interpretation of the narratives generated by participants. Frank (2010) supports a dialogical narrative analysis and discusses how this requires that the analyst "follow the storytelling" (p.104) and "enter into dialogue with a story, translating it and discovering unnoticed aspects … Interpretation is less a matter of commenting on a story than of retelling it in a varied form to create new connections" (p. 105). Frank's point is that storytelling interpretation should open up connections to more stories. We used this idea both in how the focus group participants interpreted stories and in how we interpreted the stories once transcribed.

First, extending the idea of interpretation with respect to the storytelling context itself forced us to trace conversations and how they evolved. In our focus groups, the act of telling and receiving stories required interpretation on the part of both the participant telling the story and those receiving it. We listened for ways stories were reinterpreted and led to further stories during the focus groups. Each time a story was told by a participant, we traced through the conversation and noticed the connections to other stories sometimes taking us in unexpected directions. For example, a conversation about shaving legs as a point of parental contention led to memories of makeup and a participant in that conversation extended it to implicit values and judgements from her mom, based on time and labor:

> Well, going back to the part about make-up and the shaving. That was something that was very much emphasized in my household. Between my parents, my mom was the only person working, so she was always busy there was never really time for that kind of thing. And whenever it came to makeup and shaving, I mean, I get the impression that she always thought it was kind of a frivolous thing – a sign I had too much time on my hands.
>
> -*Esther, Focus group participant*

This discussion about makeup also led Esther to discuss the role of women as caregivers and her mother in particular:

> I always got the impression that women were supposed to be stay at home moms or caregivers. It just – there's nothing wrong with being a caregiver, but there's an extent to which you care so much about everyone else that you don't have time to take care of yourself … . I mean growing up, my mom was always the one to put everybody first before herself. There would be these times when I would see her get very frustrated with that.

This idea of care for others was brought up multiple times in the focus groups – reflecting both the individual's recognition of the physical and emotional labor many women undertake in the family as well as the broader societal inequities of how much work women are expected to do in caring for children, spouses, extended family and community members. Interestingly, when we would begin the focus groups by asking about what health means to them, some participants would begin by talking about other people's health issues – often those of a spouse or someone that they had to care for – and fail to mention their own health, requiring us to steer the conversation back to their health.

In our interpretation of the stories on paper, we found new ways of thinking about them by allowing the conversations to connect across the different focus groups. Just as participants reinterpreted others' stories in telling their own, we made new connections as we interpreted the stories across the focus groups. For example, in considering the role of religion, Roseanne discussed how going to a Catholic school was the most liberal education she could have received, given how conservative her community was:

> I went to a Catholic high school … which was the most liberal thing you could do. (laughter) That's weird, but it's true … . There was no discussion of sexual health, anything like that, when I was a child, until I got to high school and then they actually had Planned Parenthood come in and do presentations. Aside from the awkward 4th grade "here are things that are going to happen to you" bits, but as far as menstrual – menstruation starting – it's kind of one of those, here are some products, take care of that, it's not something we talk about, your dad doesn't need to know it's a thing (laugh). And so, Planned Parenthood was actually the first time, they came in did a presentation and said, "ok, shake hands with your neighbors" think about how many people you talked and just touched and they talked about condoms and talked about that stuff. Which was eye opening and really good.

This story led us to consider ways that religious institutions functioned as sites of opening up sexual and reproductive health knowledge for many of our participants. Our preconceived notions of religious institutions as shutting down sexual knowledge shifted when we followed these stories across the focus groups.

A number of the participants had attended Catholic schools and they remembered that their first sex education was at these schools, sometimes from nuns. The expertise gained by one participant, Fran, at a Catholic school was later a point of pride in talking about sex with her mother:

> I actually learned about it at school. And it was taught to us by a *nun*. (laughter) Because I went to a Catholic school. They took the physiological approach to it so we at least were learning about our bodies. And I'm so remembering having to *draw* things [laughter], even having to pass the test by a hundred percent. I made a 97, it wasn't good enough. (laughter) Because they wanted to know that with a hundred percent accuracy you're walking out this door with accurate information. But I remember my mom finding my little notebook. The sex education thing, and it said A plus! … and then my sister, the older sister, was pregnant. And mom says, "You know, I'm a little worried about your sister because her sack broke 24 hours ago and the doctors are saying blah blah blah." And I said, "Well, if you look in this section, (laughter) the amniotic thing starts in a week and infection can develop, blah blah blah." "And how did you know things like that?" "Sex education."

Not everyone learned this knowledge in school, but many of our Pacific Islander participants in particular noted that sex was not discussed with them at home, only at school.

The language of sex being taught through the churches is consistent with Foucault's work on the use of discourse and power. Hopwood and colleagues (2015) summarize Foucault's perspective on communication about sex: "Language was a technology of power, exercised through the churches, the state, the schools, and the family, but silences spoke volumes, and ignorance was produced as well as knowledge" (p. 400). Although the stories our participants told with respect to what they learned at school are consistent with power, there is another way of considering the role of religion in the lives of our participants. An alternative story to be told about the role of religious education is that in addition to controlling the participants in the understanding of sex, the knowledge also gave them a place to start where they may have faltered without it.

This act of interpreting stories also requires that we take the individual's story as it is, without over-interpretation. When participants shared stories there was also a sense of how they wanted to present themselves to others, even if it may contradict other stories they tell. The ways we tell stories about ourselves may serve to reinforce or challenge what we believe about ourselves – it allows both a rethinking and a reimagining. For example, how do we think of our own sexuality and comfort with our body? One participant, Didi, despite learning to be more open about discussing the topic of sex and reproduction also considered her own discomfort with being naked:

> You know my husband still calls me prude (laughter) – I grew up Catholic, so touching is something that is like, you only touch someone behind closed doors. Or kissing in front of the public is a big no-no or holding hands. So I don't know, it's just – I'd like to be more comfortable about my own body but I just can't. I can't even take my clothes off in front of him. I tell him that we're gonna die without you seeing me naked, I'm sorry (laughter). It's just how – it's a mindset.

Yet this participant did not have trouble talking about sex and later mentioned that her sisters thought she had become Westernized because of her willingness to discuss sex. This personal conflict resonated with other participants, spurring further stories of how and when sex and body could be discussed, even with family members.

The Invisible Stories That Accompany Us

For our focus groups, we also found that participants told stories that seemed to serve as long-time "companions" in terms of shaping their beliefs about sexual and reproductive health. These stories are often invisible to others, but once shared provide an instant recognition and understanding. It is fascinating the ways such personal stories may "act" in an individual's life – holding power to shape actions across generations. Or how the personal story may serve as an "anti-story" – a reminder of why and how an individual may want to make different choices. Some of the stories were likely ones that served as "material semiotic companions" (Frank 2010). They may have been stories that represented/served as signs for making sense of life and accompanied the storyteller through time. For example, Roseanne told a story about how her mother suddenly chose to take her to get birth control:

> I had just kind of stayed away from the boys, during high school, I was a "good girl" whatever that means. And then when I left for college, though, my mom takes me to the doctor and she's like, "You need to be on the pill." So she clearly had feelings and thoughts about

> these things, but she never expressed them, never had the talk. [I]t was just so weird, that it was like "Ok, you're going to college so you need to know all this stuff now" but nothing for the first 18 years of my life.

This participant's story was one that seemed to be a "companion" as she later provided further context – her mother (who was not Asian American) had gotten pregnant in college herself. Later, this participant became a peer romance educator, gaining the knowledge she had not gotten earlier in life and she was committed to providing better information to her own children as they grew up.

The stories that are not told are constant companions for individuals too and was one challenge to overcome in terms of the resistance and discomfort we expected from participants. However, our participants clearly discussed the silence that was enforced around topics of sex in their families. We heard many stories about the kinds of statements or questions that could get you into trouble or stir memories or actions that others did not want to discuss. People create silence for a reason and that silence is crafted just as stories are. The silence carries its own power to shape choices and its influence is felt across generations. This has been discussed by other researchers, especially for the aspects of trauma not discussed in families (Dinh et al., 2018).

The absence of conversations about sex, or anything connected to the body that could be interpreted as sexual, was raised repeatedly in our focus groups. One participant recalled that not only did her mother never discuss sex, but "She wouldn't even say the word "bra" she would spell it out." Another participant, Helen, reflected on how secretiveness around sex was reinforced:

> I remember once when I was nine, my auntie and their cousins were talking about one of their cousins – they were pregnant. And I went and asked my mom, "Where do babies come from?" And she went boom (making slapping motion) slap, right here (motioning to cheek). She said, "You have to finish school." She goes, "Don't you ever ask again. You have to finish school." That's the first thing she said. And I said OK and I *never* asked again. When I went to high school, now I start learning – that's where I learned.

However, these silences were also points of cultural tradition. Helen also explained the ritual surrounding her first menstruation and how the privacy surrounding that represented a shared experience with her grandmother:

> I told my grandma and she goes, it's like – I'm going to say, almost like my birthday. She goes, "Ok, you have to go to the ocean" and

> that's when, I was over there, she put a lot of flowers around me. It was one way I got to wear flowers. Then my mom goes, "Why you wearing that?" And I don't want to tell her. It's same I don't tell my sister or my cousin. And I even told my grandma, "Do not tell nobody." It was between me and her.

On the one hand, secrecy around matters of sex is not new and is not specific to Asian American and Pacific Islander communities. However, the cultural context for how the silence was shaped reflects a contrast to ideas of shame with respect to sex. The silence around sex was related to expectations for the future, or the privacy of the act of sex between married couples. We also learned how many of our participants resisted taboos around sexual conversations is important for both the women having the conversation and the ways we think about treating them.

The focus group setting may have elicited some spur-of-the-moment stories rather than stories that had been told over and over again. In that sense, they may also have been stories that were sparked by recognition in someone else's story rather than a story that had been carefully crafted – the community space allowed a suppressed story to be shared. Such highly personal stories may serve as material semiotic companions even when they have very little structure or even when they are rarely told. Although the stories shared in our focus groups may not have been ones the participants spoke of very often, they held explanatory meaning to individuals.

Conclusion

Dan McAdams, a lifespan developmentalist, has long used life narratives in researching how people age and make sense of their lives. His theory of narrative identity focuses on how we tell our own personal stories – what choices do we make to tell our life story in a certain way? Those who can tell their life history in more integrated ways find more meaning in, and are more satisfied with, life. In fact, there is a kind of narrative therapy that helps individuals psychologically by supporting them in re-shaping their narrative identity (e.g., McAdams, 1997). Similarly, Frank (2013) in *The Wounded Storyteller* analyzes the different stories that are told of illness and the role of testimony and narrative ethics. He advocates for the importance of "thinking with stories" and listening to both one's own story and others' in detailed ways. We may be both self-reflective and generative in storytelling, helping to understand one's own circumstances but also providing ways of telling new stories for others. Frank asks, "What story do you wish to tell of yourself?. … Thinking with stories also requires attending to how a story is *used* on different occasions of its telling" (p. 159).

The shared storytelling and common narrative threads seemed to accompany participants' decisions about what they would do differently with their own children's education about sexual and reproductive health. Many recognized that the avoidance and lack of dialog, even based in cultural tradition, were not helpful. Recognizing the lessons learned from their own upbringing and wanting to change these for their children was one way of changing their stories for the future.

Using storytelling in our research has provided us with many generative ways of moving forward. We learned how storytelling transformed the research space into a community dialogue filled with recognition, advice and humor. We considered how a community focus group could be a twisted liminality, serving as an opportunity to change both researchers and participants in the process. And we have a direction forward in this work, with respect to how to present "findings" (discussed in the final chapter) and generative ways of interpreting the stories. The intimate revelations that our participants reflected in their stories may be ways of creating health revolutions in the future.

References

Andrews, N., Greenfield, S., Drever, W., & Redwood, S. (2019). Intersectionality in the liminal space: Researching Caribbean women's health in the UK context. *Frontiers in Sociology*, *4*, 82. 10.3389/fsoc.2019.00082

Baxter, V., & Low, K. E. (2017). *Applied theatre: Performing health and wellbeing*: Bloomsbury Publishing.

Bradby, H. (2017). Taking story seriously. *Social Theory & Health*, *15*(2), 206–222. 10.1057/s41285-017-0028-3

Brown, R., & Kulik, J. (1977). Flashbulb memories. *Cognition*, *5*(1), 73–99. 10.1016/0010-0277(77)90018-X

Carlson, D. L., McGuire, K., Koro, M., & Cannella, G. (2020). Twisted liminalities. *Qualitative Inquiry*, *26*(8-9), 1056–1059. 10.1177/1077800420939865

Dinh, K. T., Ho, I. K., & Tsong, Y. (2018). *Introduction to special issue: Trauma and well-being among Asian American women*. In: *Women and therapy* 41(3-4), 189-202. 10.1080/02703149.2018.1425021.

Frank, A. W. (2010). *Letting stories breathe: A socio-narratology*. University of Chicago Press.

Frank, A. W. (2013). *The wounded storyteller: Body, illness, and ethics*. University of Chicago Press.

Fraser, H. (2004). Doing narrative research: Analysing personal stories line by line. *Qualitative social work*, *3*(2), 179–201. 10.1177/1473325004043383

Garland-Thomson, R. (2005). Feminist disability studies. *Signs*, *30*(2), 1557–1587. 10.1086/423352

Hopwood, N., Jones, P. M., Kassell, L., & Secord, J. (2015). Introduction: Communicating Reproduction. *Bulletin of the History of Medicine*, *89*(3), 379. 10.1353/bhm.2015.0064

Low, K. (2017). It's difficult to talk about sex in a positive way: Creating a space to breathe. *Applied Theatre: Performing Health and Wellbeing*. Bloomsbury Methuen Drama, 146–161.

McAdams, D. P. (1997). *The stories we live by: Personal myths and the making of the self*. Guilford.
Okazaki, S. (2002). Influences of culture on Asian Americans' sexuality. *Journal of Sex Research*, *39*(1), 34–41. http://www.jstor.org/stable/3813421
Parks, P. (2023). Story circles: A new method of generative research. *American Journal of Qualitative Research*, *7*(1), 58–72. 10.29333/ajqr/12844
Turner, V. (1998). *From ritual to theatre: The human seriousness of play*. PAJ Publications.
Warren, L. (2008). *The oral tradition today: An introduction to the art of storytelling*. Pearson Custom Publishing.
Wong, G., & Breheny, M. (2018). Narrative analysis in health psychology: A guide for analysis. *Health Psychology and Behavioral Medicine*, *6*(1), 245–261. 10.1080/21642850.2018.1515017

4 Promoting Praxis

"Praxis" – according to Paulo Freire – involves "reflection and action upon the world in order to transform it" (Freire, 1972, p. 52). In this chapter, we propose seven activities involving engagement and reflection that we hope lead to actions that may begin to change our health systems for AANHPI women. The activities are proposed as a way of building community. As Freire emphasized, mutual respect and understanding are critical to the process and to creating social capital that may be harnessed for transformation. More specifically, Mvskoke scholar Laura Harjo in *Spiral to the Stars. Mvskoke Tools of Futurity* (Harjo, 2019) has identified community-building tools that have been vital to her own community's resilience, "so that we choose our future and our future does not choose us" (Harjo, 2019, p. 25). The final chapter of her book provides a series of "methods" that "can provide opportunities for individuals and communities to realize their own power and agency" (Harjo, 2019, p. 47). Harjo's example inspired us to include this final chapter of activities in the hopes of encouraging AANHPI women to reflect upon their own experiences and to empower themselves as the authorities about their own health and health needs. These activities also support the process of "unveiling" the ways that past stories, the ones we tell ourselves and the ones imposed upon us (especially those connected to race, gender, culture, and immigrant heritage) influence the health of AANHPI women.

We have imagined that AANHPI women and/or AANHPI community members will participate in these activities. These activities, however, may also be scaled to specific ethnic communities with specific shared histories. We suggest conferring with a community member who is well acquainted with the target participants to ensure that the wording will be accessible based on diversity of education and English fluency. However, we also recognize that some of these activities could be used to inform health care professionals, and thus suggest that some of these activities may be adapted so that HCPs might gain a sense of what

DOI: 10.4324/9781003449867-5

AANHPI women with different levels of English fluency, trust levels, and education might experience or may anticipate based on previous social interactions. Some of these activities may simply be a way to start conversations about AANHPI women's health or interactions with HCPs. Other activities may be more about building a sense of community by starting with low-risk involvement such as warm-up activities that emphasize engagement. These can help break the ice by having participants all participate and feel more comfortable with each other and the activities.

Organizing Meetings with AANHPI Women and Community Members

Before one works with AANHPI women and members of the AANHPI community to address women's health, the organization or individual must first do some work and outreach. Because the authors already had a history with local community organizations, we were able to draw upon our connections to organize our focus groups. Even so, we still relied upon community members who had worked with some of the communities we did not know ourselves. One community member, for example, explained to us the specific way one community was organized, and how formal leaders in the community must be approached with information about our project and goals. If the leaders did not give permission, we would not be able to recruit any of the community members because they would not participate. This is an example of learning the specific protocols and social organization of the community and showing respect to the process acknowledged within the community itself. If we did not already have relationships with community organizations, we would have had to start by doing research by identifying members of the community who might in turn be able to connect us to community leaders. Other resources include identifying ethnic organizations and reading ethnic-specific media.

Several years earlier, when our academic program developed a report about AANHPIs in our state (APAZI, 2006), we even ate at local restaurants to connect with recent Burmese immigrants as well as the local Tongan community. We introduced ourselves and made casual conversation. Over time, as we built relationships and ate delicious food, we were able to ask about the larger community. In one instance, the couple did not know of a larger community. In the other, we were able to organize a community gathering at the restaurant to ask community members about the issues they found most pressing in relation to their community at that time. However, in the latter case, because we did not sustain those relationships (the community leader we worked with ended up moving from the area) we were not able to call upon those connections with the current AANHPI women's sexual health project. In other cases, however, team members had sustained relationships with community organizations and were able to draw upon that organization to send out an email call for participants for a focus group. Demonstrating a desire for ongoing relations with the community may include attending and participating in fundraising events, community fairs or activities, and contributing one's time. Because our academic program regularly has participated in the local Matsuri festival for example, we even recruited some focus group participants by setting up an interactive activity at our booth.

Community Diversity

Although community is often viewed as positive, sometimes community norms may be a limiting factor to how much women are willing to share about their sexual and reproductive health. It is important to be cognizant of the great diversity within AANHPI communities, and to recognize that caste status and socioeconomic status are factors within some AANHPI communities as they are in other communities. Differences of religion, caste, socioeconomic status, political ideology, familial affiliations, and/or sexuality may contribute to the silencing of some women in gatherings, just as these differences contribute to the silencing of some women in their own communities. Ethnic differences among AANHPI women also may lead to discomfort and are important to understand. Thus, it's important to work with community members who value the project and perceive (or even suggest) ways in which it may benefit their communities; often they will know some of the nuances of internal community politics, traditional hierarchies, and the correct protocols to engage community participation.

Additionally, key community members at times may be formal leaders, and at times may be individuals who informally lead by assisting others in the community. Women often may not be identified as formal community leaders but may be identified as key community members. Of course, communities feature multiple networks with different individuals who carry influence in specific networks. Identifying these key people can make the difference in successfully recruiting a range of participants to attend your events. And some women, depending on culture and generation, may not feel comfortable communicating with strangers, particularly those of the opposite sex. When developing communication and conversation, it is always important to ask the participants themselves to identify key issues. A formal leader may not be aware of the gendered or classed (for example) differences in experiences and perceptions. Importantly, when working with community partners, it is vital to hear and respond to their concerns. During an event that a prominent community leader attended, we chose to change our presentation after asking a community member about whether a cultural reference would be problematic (it did not relate to sexual health). While some academics might question this decision, our concern was to ensure that our community partner would continue to have a positive relationship with this community leader. Including content that makes sense for academic audiences does not always translate in community settings and could jeopardize the effectiveness of our partner's community outreach.

One of the challenges of working with AANHPI communities is the diversity of languages possible. In areas with larger communities, it may be possible to designate some meetings as Mandarin-speaking or Tagalog-speaking. However, in smaller communities, there may be a range of languages and fluencies, and if there are no translator services (including sign language) or volunteers (often family members of individuals) then the groups will self-select with those who communicate in English. Asian Immigrant Workers Advocates (AIWA), an Oakland, California-based non-profit organization, works regularly with immigrant women and seeks to include translators at every event. If resources permit, providing translators is an important way to host inclusive events. AIWA also encourages women to communicate in the language they feel most comfortable with at their meetings, even if this takes longer with the accompanying translation both of what some women communicate and to translate what is communicated to women who may be fluent in other languages (Shin, 2010). This is an important consideration when organizing an event.

Who Is Invited? Who May Participate?

When organizing a meeting of AANHPI women to discuss sexual and reproductive health, certain concerns must be considered, including the communities' own definitions and expectations which may reflect differences of age, generation, religion, and so forth. For example, not every community member may agree on the definition of who is a woman. Not all AANHPI communities agree on a common definition; there may be generational differences about transgender, intersex, or gender fluid individuals.

When it comes to organizing focus groups, understanding the specific community dynamics and norms may require organizing focus groups based on ethnicity, sexuality, generation and/or age, or religion. With larger community meetings, this may mean making very clear both in outreach materials and at the outset of the meeting the definitions that the organizers are using to define AANHPI women to avoid any misunderstandings of conflict: does this include multiracial women of AANHPI heritage and/or transgender women, are men invited to attend and participate in discussions, would parents be comfortable if their children are present for all the discussions, and so forth.

If this is a meeting of health care providers to discuss best practices working with AANHPI women, the presence of health care workers of AANHPI heritage means taking care that facilitators or participants do NOT expect those participants to represent the whole of their culture or heritage. It also means taking care should someone claim to speak from authority about AANHPI culture or health or experiences that what is said is not generalized to represent entire communities. One way to address both scenarios (AANHPI community gatherings or HCP gatherings) is to identify common understandings for discussion and participation that emphasize the value of individual experience, acknowledge the social structures, values, and differences within the community, and do not place undue expectations on individuals to speak on behalf of an entire community or category of persons within a community. For example, one understanding may be: "When people speak, we understand that they are speaking from their own perspectives, knowledge, and experience and not speaking for an entire community or group." Another may be, "When asking someone a question, we understand that they are not being asked to represent anyone's perspectives or experiences other than their own." A particularly important understanding that may be reiterated verbally is, "We value all participants today for the knowledge they bring from their own experiences; we want to hear from everyone who wishes to contribute. If anyone is uncomfortable speaking up, we invite them to write down their thoughts and provide them to a facilitator." This understanding needs to be confirmed through active listening and lack of interruption on the part of the facilitators hosting the meeting.

The University of Kansas Center for Community Health and Development has an online Community Tool Box that provides resources for those working with communities, building community networks, and navigating different situations. It has 46 chapters focusing on specific skill sets related to building community (See https://ctb.ku.edu/en).

Hospitality

Providing refreshments for gatherings is an effective way to demonstrate hospitality and appreciation when one invites community members to participate in an in-person focus group or meeting. Putting out bottled water and fresh fruit, along with napkins, is a simple way to demonstrate appreciation. Items with peanuts are best avoided due to common food allergies.

Closing the Meeting

How one ends the meeting is just as important as how one begins – with gratitude and appreciation, and with specific explanations of the next steps either for the community or for the project and either how the community members will be updated or may opt in to stay informed. While providing a space to address challenges and concerns has been described by participants in our study as valuable, addressing these challenges may also be difficult. It is important to end the meeting on an empowering note, and to provide a list of community resources for support and continued engagement for participants if possible.

Note: The following activities are designed when meeting with AANHPI women and/or AANHPI community members. If having a meeting primarily with healthcare providers, we recommend shifting the activities to place the HCPs in the position of understanding what it would be like to experience such interactions – being treated as an outsider, assuming one does not speak English, and so forth.

Activities

Activity 1: Changing Representations: What Does it Mean to be an AANHPI Woman

As the introduction and chapter 1 illustrated, the ways in which AANHPI women think about themselves are shaped by broader society and the ways that policies, social values, media, and history have constructed them. This compares with the cultural messages received from their immediate family and community, creating spaces for alternative and different experiences and ideas.

If you are working with college-educated second or later generation AANHPI women who have English fluency, you might have a discussion about a common reading. *Suggested readings*: Nellie Wong (1981) "When I was Growing Up" or M. Evelina Galang (1996) "The Look Alike Women." Note: We suggest encouraging participants to identify additional poems or short pieces to share with others for discussion. While Wong writes from a Chinese American perspective and Galang from a Filipina perspective, these pieces speak across ethnic identities about the cultural expectations placed on women in the United States.

- Ask participants to read either or both pieces ahead of discussion, and to reflect upon their own experiences with the following questions. (Note: Asian and NHPI are racial categories; Japanese, Thai, Cambodian, Pakistani, Indian, CHamoru, Kānaka Maoli, are examples of ethnicities.)

  Can you identify with any of the messages the women in the readings received about being women?
  How did these messages make you feel about yourself?

If you are working with a group that may not be comfortable reading the short pieces, you may simply ask the participants to share when they have felt they stood out because they were Asian American and/or Pacific Islander women, and why. Then ask other participants if they had similar experiences. Then ask, "How did you respond?" And end by asking, "How do you wish you responded?" to allow participants to think of alternate, possibly more empowering responses.

Activity 2: Dissecting the Details: Addressing Microaggressions

Many AANHPIs have experienced the sting of offhand comments related to their race and gender. These comments differ from direct insults or attacks because they often seem unintentional or minor (hence "micro") but may cause just as much hurt. Derald Wing Sue defined these experiences as *microaggressions* (Sue, 2021). The facilitator may wish to view/listen to Sue's talk, "Microaggressions in Everyday Life" on YouTube or, if it is accessible to the group, watch/listen to the 15-minute video together first. This activity is an opportunity to acknowledge and discuss these experiences, categorize them as the different types of microaggressions and generate community and individual responses to microaggressions. This activity is meant to be energizing and validating to those participants who may have experienced microaggressions but not categorized them in that way.

- Go over what constitutes a microaggression: unlike direct negative comments, microaggressions may be framed as compliments, offhand observations, or casual actions. These actions, however, reveal negative assumptions that are insulting, harmful. Thus, these often unintentional forms of prejudice are called "microaggressions."

Discuss a couple of prominent examples – "Where are you from?" which may convey that one is perceived as an outsider. "You speak good English" communicates an expectation that the person would not be fluent in English because they are seen as foreign. "Are you really Asian?" might suggest that only persons of East Asian ancestry are considered Asian.

- Ask individuals or groups to come up with as many examples as possible and write them down on a whiteboard or piece of paper.
- Discuss these examples of microaggressions. Possible prompts may be: Do any of these statements or actions sound familiar to you? How do they make you feel?

- As a whole group, discuss possible responses. These may be on a community level (community-level campaigns to address racial microaggressions) or individual level (responses/actions for the moment when the microaggression occurs; see Boal section below as an idea about practicing these responses). It takes practice to be prepared to respond in the moment, so consider a range of responses, from short remarks to longer explanations.

Activity 3: Storytelling Circles: Belonging and Acceptance

In one large group, invite everyone in the circle to share in response to storytelling prompts. An individual may choose to pass, but no questions or comments are made between stories. The purpose of the process is for individuals to have the opportunity to share a story without judgment; the only restriction may be time limitations for each participant. Once everyone in the circle has had the opportunity to share their story, the moderator may ask for reflections. Some suggested prompts:

- Recall a specific time when you felt you belonged. Who was there? Where did it happen? What made you feel that you belonged?

  What specific places do you feel as if you belong or are accepted? What are the actions of others that help you to feel welcome and accepted?

- Recall a specific time you felt you were not welcome or accepted. What led to this feeling? Who was there?

  What kinds of places feel less welcoming or accepting? What do others do that promotes a feeling of non-acceptance?

- What experiences with healthcare professionals or in medical settings helped you feel accepted and heard?
- What experiences with healthcare professionals or in medical settings felt unwelcoming?

Follow-up questions after storytelling:

- Have these actions ever made you feel as if you don't want to seek out health care?
- When you do not feel welcome or not accepted, who do you turn to?
- What actions can/should we take to change/respond to the medical system?

Activity 4: Humor in Health

In our focus groups, we were surprised at the amount of laughter and humor that was shared while recounting stories of learning about sexual intimacy, menstruation, and reproduction. Prompts asking for participants to recount their first memories of learning about sex and when they started their period provided details about cultural differences and practices and funny interactions with family members. The lighter atmosphere in the focus groups led us to work with performance artist Kristina Wong for a community event where we discussed our research project and Wong led the audience through activities and told stories about her own experiences relating to sexual and reproductive health. The event included opportunities for attendees to depict their own relationship to sex and reproduction through paper folding and storytelling.

- Generate opportunities to share memories through some of the following prompts:

  When did you first hear the word sex? How did you learn about it? Who did you talk with?
  What was it like when you started your period? How old were you? Where were you?
  What conversations did you have with family members about sex and reproduction?

- If you had to represent sex through a piece of paper, what would it look like? Kristina Wong (https://www.kristinawong.com/about/) designed this activity for our workshop: she gave everyone a piece of paper; some people smushed the paper up, some ripped it, some folded it into a shape, some wrote on it.

Activity 5: Understanding What It Means to Be Heard and Acknowledged

These questions are meant to open up discussion. We recommend only choosing a few to break the ice and having a few ready as potential follow-up questions.

- Have there been any cases where you feel your loved ones do not pay attention to your input or that you are not being acknowledged?
- What does that feel like?
- How do you show your loved ones that you are paying attention to them and care about them?
- How do you show people that you may not know that you are paying attention to their perspective?

Understanding what it means to not be understood or not acknowledged.

- Have you ever been ignored or dismissed at a business or in a social setting? How did that make you feel?
- What did you do to be acknowledged?

Understanding power dynamics in your everyday life

- Have you ever felt scrutinized or the focus of attention? How many times are you highly aware of others and why?
- Have you ever felt ignored? Why do you think you were being ignored?
- Have you ever been asked to repeat yourself? How many times did you ask others to repeat themselves and why?
- Has anyone ever spoken loudly to you as if you could not understand? When have you done so with others and why?
- Have you ever experienced having your individual actions interpreted as representing all other people who look like you? Why do you think this was the case? How did it make you feel? Have there been times you have done so with others? How might you stop yourself from making certain assumptions about others?
- Have you ever worried that your actions might be misinterpreted in a negative way and why?
- Did you ever think that you might be perceived as being out of place and why?
- Describe a situation where you were aware of being different than others around you. How did you respond to this situation?

For any of the above questions: What actions might you take to change any of these interactions?

For example, one way that women have supported each other in meetings is to reiterate what each other has said, particularly when that person's contribution is ignored and then repeated by a participant who may enjoy a privileged position in that setting, who then gets credit. Another woman who notices this might speak up, "I agree with Person B (person in privileged position). Person A (who stated original idea) suggested this earlier, and it's great idea." This means paying attention to whose work and contributions may go unacknowledged in organizations and places of work for various reasons and affirming their contributions. This kind of allyship can create community and reciprocity for each other.

Activity 6: Empowerment through Action

Because some activities ask participants to reflect on negative experiences, we suggest closing with this activity or another that is uplifting.

This exercise draws upon concepts from Augusto Boal's *Theatre of the Oppressed* (Boal & McBride 1985) to enact responses to microaggressions, being ignored, or invalidated. Some of Boal's activities allow those who have experienced a feeling of powerlessness (being ignored or being talked down to) to respond to these situations in a space with supportive people. This may provide participants with ideas for responding when similar actions occur and may help participants gain the confidence and skills of responding with power. While this activity is simplified, some organizations may find people trained in this kind of approach who are willing to facilitate the activity. For a longer set of activities and ideas, we found that Gopal Midha's "Theater of the Oppressed a Manual for Educators" (Midha, 2010) online provided excellent exercises.

First, ask participants to sit in a circle (not a U) so that they can see each other. The facilitator should always be on the same level as the participants, sitting or standing. If some participants are not able to stand, then it would be good for all participants to sit on chairs (as some may not be able to sit on the floor). If the group has been sitting for a while or unengaged, we recommend beginning with one warm-up exercise before the activity.

Ask the group: Have you ever had any negative or uncomfortable experiences in the doctor's office? List responses on a whiteboard/large piece of paper posted on the wall. Identify the most common experience. Ask volunteers (arrange beforehand in case) to enact the scenario with the doctor/patient or the receptionist/patient or other patients/patient. Then ask volunteers to switch places and enact a different response that counters the action, microaggression, or exchange.

Warm up Exercises: (choose one): Boal practitioners often encourage warm up exercises to get people moving and feel more at ease in role-playing or acting out responses. Here are a few:

Elbow to Elbow (BusyTeacher.org, 2018). Have participants stand in the middle of the room. After the facilitator calls out an attribute (City of residence, Favorite book, Tennis Shoe brand, etc.), participants will link elbows or otherwise convey a connection with another person who shares the same attribute (limit of two persons per someone with attribute). If not enough folks fit that attribute, that's okay, just call out another attribute. This will not work for folks who do not speak the same language.

Would you rather? (BusyTeacher.org, 2018) Ask a series of questions – would you rather be a butterfly or a dragonfly? Would you rather bowl or fish? Divide the room into two sides and point to each side. Those who agree with one identity will move to that side or the other. Those who are not able to easily move may be asked to indicate in a different way.

Random acts of description (not suited if some participants cannot move their limbs): Ask the participants to enact random words (e.g., avocado, rice cooker, blender, car) – and then move from random words to words relating to health (health, wellness, joy, energy, strength).

What fills your bucket: (Michigan, 2021) What fills your bucket? What drains you? What do you value most about what you have to offer when you feel your best energy?

Note: Additional ideas may be found with an online search, with attention paid to inclusivity for those who may not be fluent in English or U.S. culture or may have physical or mental disabilities.

Activity 7 (adapted from **Open in Emergency***: A Special Issue on Asian American Mental Health (Khúc, 2016))*

Although this book has focused on AANHPI women's sexual and reproductive health, we recognize that ongoing attention to overall wellness, including mental and emotional well-being is necessary. In 2016, Mimi Khúc, Ph.D., editor of the *Asian American Literary Review*, curated a series of activities with other Asian American scholars, *Open in Emergency: A Special Issue on Asian American and Mental Health.* One activity consisted of a deck of Asian American tarot cards that could be used to open up conversations about external expectations, internalized pressures, and overall wellness. A pamphlet about postpartum depression included edits by Asian Americans who had experienced postpartum depression themselves and demystified the condition along with the pressures new mothers face. The pamphlet could facilitate discussion about the experience, idealized motherhood, and counter the ways fears and feelings might be minimized by others. This "emergency kit" has been used in classrooms and community groups to prompt discussion and reflection on the part of participants (Hiscott, 2019). Unfortunately, it is not available at this time. Instead, we suggest one or two possible ways to incorporate Khúc's approach to opening up discussions about wellness:

A Screen Khúc's Ted Talk, The Revolution is in the Heart, at https://youtu.be/3mBRcSH5IHY (approximately 17 minutes). Facilitators may preview this talk and prepare a few open-ended questions about feelings, being human, and wellness.

B Mimi Khúc also offers workshops and dialogs in a variety of formats (including virtual). Please see her website to learn more about the types of workshops and presentations she offers: https://www.mimikhuc.com/booking

C Several AANHPI organizations that focus on mental health suggest activities for balance, mindfulness, and wellness. Please see Appendix B for a list of selected organizations and their websites. Some groups already linked through affinity (in the case of our focus groups, several participants were members of ethnic and religious organizations) sponsor group activities. The JACL AZ women's group for example holds cooking classes where different generations cook together. These focused activities in community may also promote a sense of well-being.

Activity 8. Ask the Other Question: Understanding Interconnectedness

Mari Matsuda, the first tenured female Asian American law professor in the United States, has written about the importance of Asian Americans supporting social justice for everyone, not simply Asian Americans. She frequently has questioned the model minority stereotype that positions Asian Americans more favorably in relation to other communities of color, using selective, visible examples of Asian American economic and academic success to suggest other communities of color somehow don't work hard enough (Matsuda, 1993). She also has called upon Asian Americans to be accountable to social justice by practicing solidarity and building coalitions with other groups facing systemic discrimination, including the act of acknowledging how Asian Americans may benefit from the subordination of others even as Asian Americans also face subordination (Matsuda, 1991). In this latter discussion, "Beside My Sister, Facing the Enemy: Legal Theory Out of Coalition," Matsuda describes moments of discomfort she has felt, at one point expressing a microaggression against a Black feminist scholar, and another as a Japanese American whose family migrated to work in Hawai`i when hearing Native Hawaiian Haunani-Kay Trask critiquing the dispossession of Native Hawaiians of their lands – a dispossession that has benefitted Asian Americans and others who now call Hawai`i home. Matsuda states, "I could shelter myself from conflict by leaving the conversation, but I have come to believe that the comfort we feel when we avoid hard conversations is a dangerous comfort, one that seduces us into ignorance about the experiences of others and about the full meaning of our own lives." (1185–1186).

After explaining coalition – working together across differences to make structural change happen – Matsuda explains how she tries to become more aware of "the interconnection of all forms of subordination … through a method I call 'ask the other question.' When I see something that looks racist, I ask, 'Where is the patriarchy in this?' When I see something that looks sexist, I ask, "Where is the heterosexism in this?" (Matsuda, 1991, 1189; see also Davis et al., 2022, 3). This method reinforces for her how all forms of subordination intersect.

- Depending on the group and timeline, present our summary of Matsuda's method, or read either of Matsuda's essays, "We Will Not Be Used" 1993" or "Beside My Sister. Facing the Enemy" (1991), and review Matsuda's method.

- Ask the Other Question. Again, depending on available time, facilitators may draw upon activities earlier in this chapter to identify issues of concern to the participants, or facilitators may prepare cards with easily identifiable topics ahead of time (e.g. "Anti-AANHPI Hate Acts," "Immigrant rights") and ask participants: what is the other question? (thinking about where are class interests; the settler colonial interests – the interests of non-Indigenous settlers who have benefitted from colonization; the Indigenous interests; the heterosexism or homophobia; transphobia; anti-Blackness; ableism; and so forth, in this issue).
- After discussing the other questions for an issue, discuss what it would look like to build coalitions with other groups, both within the AANHPI community and beyond the AANHPI community. This might lead to discussion about the ways social structures have been set up to divide marginalized groups against each other. The 2021 COVID-19 Hate Crimes Act (popularly known as the Anti-Asian Hate Crimes Act) increased crime reporting and relied on policing to address anti-Asian violence during the pandemic. This bill, however, also further contributes to the ongoing policing of Black and Brown communities (Davis et al., 2022) and does not address the larger structural issues of lack of mental health care that may be a factor (Yam, 2021). By not asking the other questions, this seeming solution may create greater harm to communities of color. For more information about Asian American – Black relations, we suggest reading Demsas and Ramirez, 2021.
- This activity also may be varied. One might identify specific issues affecting other groups and ask how it affects one's own group. Allyship does not mean that one should always look for one's own interests in other's issues. However, understanding how one group's disadvantage might advantage one's own group interest is just as important to solidarity and coalition building as understanding how one shares disadvantages with other groups. This is also the case within AANHPI communities. A good example of the former is where Matsuda cites Haunani-Kay Trask reminding settlers in Hawai`i, which include Asian Americans, that their presence is due to the overthrow of the Hawaiian monarchy and the dispossession of Native Hawaiians (Trask, 1991).

  An example of the latter is when Arizona's state law SB1070 promoted racial surveillance of those perceived to not be "legal immigrants." Even though this bill clearly supported police surveillance of Latinx Americans, some South Asians and other Asian Americans reported being asked to show documents demonstrating their legal status in the United States. Assumptions that tattoos denote gang activity also have justified police surveillance of certain bodies, and Pacific Islanders who may have tattoos for cultural significance have been targeted for police scrutiny. Historical examples of forced sterilization of women of color, especially Native American, Black, and Latinx women, may be compared to the ways that Asian immigrant communities had their second generations delayed because of restrictions on the immigration of Asian women (see Miliann Kang, as cited in Chapter 1).

References

APAZI. (2006). *The State of Asian Americans and Pacific Islanders in Arizona*. Retrieved from Tempe, AZ: https://keep.lib.asu.edu/items/141108

Boal, A., & McBride, M.-O. L. (1985). Theatre of the Oppressed. In *The Applied Theatre Reader* (pp. 134–140). Routledge.

BusyTeacher.org. (2018). 6 Fun and Simple Games to Help your Shy Students. Retrieved from https://m.busyteacher.org/23613-shy-students-6-fun-simple-games.html

Davis, A.Y., Dent, G., Meiners, E.R., & Richie, B.E. (2022). *Abolition. Feminism. Now*. Haymarket Books.

Demsas, J. & Ramirez, R. (2021). The history of tensions – and solidarity – between Black and Asian communities, explained. *Vox*. Retrieved from https://www.vox.com/22321234/black-asian-american-tensions-solidarity-history

Freire, P. (1972). Education: domestication or liberation? *Prospects*, *2*(2), 173–181.

Galang, E. (1996). *Her Wild American Self*. Coffee House.

Harjo, L. (2019). *Spiral to the stars: Mvskoke tools of futurity*. University of Arizona Press.

Hiscott, R. (2019). "Open in Emergency" Explores the Asian American Mental Health Crisis — and Offers New Tools for Care. Retrieved from https://medium.com/kickstarter/open-in-emergency-explores-the-asian-american-mental-health-crisis-and-offers-new-tools-for-ca78c7cb685d

Khúc, M. (2016). *Open in emergency: A special issue on Asian American mental health*. Washington, DC: Asian American Literary Review.

Matsuda, M. (1991). Beside my sister, facing the enemy: Legal theory out of coalition. *Stanford Law Review*, *43*(6), 1183–1192.

Matsuda, M. (1993). We Will Not Be Used. *Asian American Pacific Islands Law Journal*, *1*(1), 79–84.

Michigan Department of Education. (2021). Various Ideas for Introductory Activities and Energizers. Retrieved from https://www.michigan.gov/documents/ltc/Introductory_Activities_and_Energizers_Various_Options_for_._320957_7.pdf

Midha, G. (2010). *Theatre of the oppressed A manual for educators*. Retrieved from https://scholarworks.umass.edu/cgi/viewcontent.cgi?article=1010&context=cie_capstons

Shin, Y. (2010). What does it take for limited-English speaking immigrant women to participate meaningfully in the broader society? *KALW News*. Retrieved from https://www.aiwa.org/wp-content/uploads/2014/08/KALW_News_0410.pdf

Sue, D. W. (2021). Microaggressions: death by a thousand cuts. *Scientific American*. Retrieved from https://www.scientificamerican.com/article/microaggressions-death-by-a-thousand-cuts/

Trask, H.-K. (1991). Lovely hula hands: Corporate tourism and the prostituion of Hawaiian Culture. *Border/Lines*, *23*(Winter), 22–29. Retrieved from https://journals.lib.unb.ca/index.php/bl/article/view/24958/28913

Wong, N. (1981). When I Was Growing Up. In C. Moraga & G. Anzaldúa (Eds.), *This bridge called my back: writings by radical wormen of color*. San Francisco, CA: Aunt Lute Book Company.
Yam, K. (2021). Why over 85 Asian American, LGBTQ groups opposed the anti-Asian hate crimes bill. *NBC News*. Retrieved from https://www.nbcnews.com/news/asian-america/why-over-85-asian-american-lgbtq-groups-opposed-anti-asian-n1267421

Appendix A
Focus Group Script and Survey

Project Title: Sexual and Reproductive Health and Well-being among Asian American and Pacific Islander Women in Arizona

Research Focus Group Script

Introduction

Hello and welcome to this focus group discussion. My name is [insert name] and I am here working as the facilitator/moderator. I am working on a research study with my colleagues (Professors Aggie J. Noah, Kathy Nakagawa, and Karen J. Leong,) at Arizona State University. My role is to help get a conversation going and to make sure we cover a number of important topics that they would like your input on.

1. Introduction – Purpose

First, I would like to thank you all for taking time out of your day to come here and to share your stories. The overall goal is to hear your thoughts about how we think and feel about sexual and reproductive health, and how they are related to your own experiences.

In particular, we are interested in your views about: (1) what "health" means to you, (2) what sexual and reproductive health means to you, and (3) what are some places that are important to you when you think about (sexual and reproductive) health.

We are asking you because you have identified yourself as Asian American or Pacific Islander women. Although Asian Americans are the fastest growing racial group in the United States, the unique experiences of Asian American and Pacific Islanders are not well understood in health research.

Explaining the purpose for setting up the focus group meeting:

You are the experts and we are here to learn from you;
This is strictly voluntary and you can stop your participation at any given time;

You can choose to not answer any of the questions we may ask without explaining why; and

I will be recording audio when the group discussion starts. We are recording audio so that we do not miss anything important you share and so that we can go back and revisit the information later if we want to.

2. Housekeeping

The total length of time of the focus group meeting is expected to be about one hour and a half. As far as the focus groups are concerned, there are a few "ground rules":

I might move you along in conversation. Since we have limited time, I will ask that questions or comments of the topic be answered after the focus group session.

I would like to hear everyone speak so I might ask people who have not spoken up to comment.

Please respect each other's opinions. There is no right or wrong answer to any questions I will ask. We want to hear what each of you think and it is okay to have different opinions.

We would like to stress that we want to keep the sessions confidential so we ask that you not use names or anything directly identifying when you talk about your personal experiences. We also ask that you not discuss other participants' responses outside of the discussion. However, because this is in a group setting, the other individuals participating will know your responses to the questions and we cannot guarantee that they will not discuss your responses outside of the focus group.

3. Consent Forms

Do you have any questions so far? Again your participation here today is totally voluntary. So if you are okay with moving forward, we would like to get your consent. Please take the time to review the consent form and ask any questions and/or concerns you might have. If you decide not to participate or do not want to participate, please feel free to leave. [After the first written consent form is collected] Thank you for agreeing to be part of the study. Please take the time to review the interview release form and ask any questions and/or concerns you might have.

4. Focus Group Research Questions

There are many ways people think and feel about health. We would like to hear about how you think and feel about health and how your own unique experiences make you think and feel about health (particularly your immigration experience):

What does "health" mean to you? How do you feel about your own health?
What does "sexual and reproductive health" mean to you? How do you feel about your own sexual and reproductive health?
How did you learn about sexual health? What was the first conversation you remember having about sexual health?
How did you learn about health when you were growing up? Was sexual health part of conversations about health?
What kinds of expectations did your parents have about sex? Did they ever talk to you about their expectations?
When you were growing up, was sex considered a part of everyday life, or was it something people didn't talk about? What words come to mind when you hear the word "sex"?
What attitudes did your parents teach you about health? What did your family associate with health (e.g., doctors, lifestyle, diet)? What did you learn about health from your family? Did your mother talk with you about sexual health? If not, who did you talk to?
When you think about your own sexual and reproductive health, what are some places that have been important to you? (When we say "place", it could refer to your own home, neighborhood, and other places like a hospital or friends' house – both in the United States and other places in your home country).

5. Wrapping Up

I think we have come to the end of our questions. Let me be the first to say thank you for your honest opinions – you were tremendously helpful at this very early, but very important stage of this research. As the second and last part of your participation, please fill out this survey. Taking the survey should take about 10-15 minutes.

Again, thank you very much for your participation today. We really appreciate your help. If you have any questions or concerns about the research and/or your participation, please feel free to contact Professors Aggie J. Noah, Kathy Nakagawa, and Karen J. Leong at Arizona State University. Here is their contact information:

Dr. Aggie J. Noah	Aggie.Noah@asu.edu
Dr. Kathy Nakagawa	nakagawa@asu.edu
Dr. Karen J. Leong	Karen.Leong@asu.edu

Post-Interview Survey

NOTE: The survey includes the questions as used in our project. However, we would recommend revising and expanding the questions to eliminate the heteronormative bias.

Introduction

As the second and last part of your participation, please fill out this survey. Taking the survey should take about 10-15 minutes. It is important that you answer questions honestly, but you do not have to answer any questions that you are uncomfortable completing. Thank you for your study participation.

Thank you very much for sharing your knowledge and for your honest opinions. We really appreciate your help, and your stories are very important to us. If you have any questions or concerns about the research and/or your participation, please feel free to contact Professors Aggie J. Noah, Kathy Nakagawa, and Karen J. Leong at Arizona State University. Here is their contact information:

Dr. Aggie J. Noah	Aggie.Noah@asu.edu
Dr. Kathy Nakagawa	nakagawa@asu.edu
Dr. Karen J. Leong	Karen.Leong@asu.edu

1. Basic Socioeconomic and Demographic Questions

1 Which group best describes your national origin? (Please choose one)

1 Asian Indian/South Asian
2 Chinese
3 Filipino
4 Japanese
5 Korean
6 Vietnamese
7 Other Asian – Please specify: ______________________
8 Hawaiian
9 Guamanian
10 Samoan
11 Other Pacific Islander – Please specify: __________________

2 How old are you? ______________________ years old
3 Were you born in the United States?

1 Yes
2 No

If you were not born in the United States, what year did you move to the United States? ___________

4 What year did you move to Arizona? ________________________
5 How much school did you complete?

0 None
1 1 to 11 Grades (Grades 1 through 11)
2 High School Graduate or Equivalent (e.g., GED)
3 Some College
4 Associate's Degree (AA)
5 Bachelor's Degree (BA, BS)
6 Graduate or Professional School (After Completing College)

6 Are you currently working?

1 Yes
2 No

7 What is your occupation at this job? ________________________

2. Family and Relationship Questions

B1 What is your current marital status?

1 Currently Married
2 Not Married, but Living with a Partner
3 Separated
4 Widowed
5 Divorced
6 Never Married

B2 If currently married or living with a partner, how many years have you been together? ________________________ years
B3 Do you have any children?

1 Yes
2 No

B4 Please indicate gender and age of all your children:

# of Children	Gender	Age
Child # 1		
Child # 2		
Child # 3		
Child # 4		

(*Continued*)

Child # 5		
Child # 6		
Child # 7		
Child # 8		
Child # 9		
Child # 10		

3. General Health Questions

1 Think about your health. Would you say your health in general is excellent, very good, good, fair or poor?

1 Excellent
2 Very Good
3 Good
4 Fair
5 Poor

2 Is there a place that you usually go to when you are sick or need advice about your health?

0 No, I do not have a place I usually go to
1 Clinic, Health Center or HMO
2 Doctor's Office
3 Hospital Emergency Room
4 Hospital Outpatient Department
5 Some Other Place – Please specify: ____________________

3 What is the name of this place? ________________________
4 Where is this place located? What street is it on? What is the nearest cross-street? What city is it in?

On ________________________ (Street)
Near ________________________ (Cross-Street)
In ____________________ (City) ____________________ (State)

5 Is that the same place you usually go when you need routine or preventive care, such as physical examination or check up?

1 Yes
2 No
3 No, I do not do routine or preventive care

4. Sexual Health Questions

1 Are you currently using any types of contraception or any method of preventing pregnancy?

1 Yes
2 No
3 Not currently sexually active; No contraception needed

2 Please tell us what method or methods are you using? (Check all that apply):

1 Condom (Rubber)
2 Foam, Jelly, Cream, Sponge, Suppositories
3 Withdrawal (Pulling Out)
4 Diaphragm (With or Without Jelly)
5 Rhythm (Safe Time, Avoiding Sex at Certain Times of the Month)
6 Birth Control Pills
7 IUD (Intrauterine Device)
8 Norplant, Depo-Provera or Injectables
9 Partner/Spouse has had operation/vasectomy/sterilization
10 Method not listed above – Please specify: ________________

3 When you have any concerns and/or questions about your sexual health, who would you likely talk to first?:

1 No One
2 Medical Professional (Doctor, Nurse)
3 Partner/Spouse (including Girlfriend/Boyfriend)
4 Friends
5 Siblings (Sisters, Brothers)
6 Parents
7 Coworkers
8 Other – Please specify: ______________________

5. Interview Focus Group Follow-Up Questions

During the interview and/or focus group conversation, you mentioned a place(s) that have been important to you when you think about your own sexual and reproductive health. We would like to ask you some questions about the place(s) you mentioned. We understand that answering these questions can be difficult. You can answer the questions to your best recollection and do not have to fill out every question. For example, if you only remember the city and country of a place, you can only provide that information. You can also ask the researcher in sight to ask any questions.

[PLACE 1]

1 What type of a place is this? (e.g., friend's house, doctor's office, etc.) ______________________________
2 What is the name of this place, if any? ______________________
3 Where is this place located? What street is it on? What is the nearest cross-street? What city is it in? What COUNTRY is it in?

On ______________________ (Street)
Near ______________________ (Cross-Street)
In ____________________ (City) __________________ (State)
In ______________________ (Country)

[PLACE 2]

1 What type of a place is this? (e.g., friend's house, doctor's office, etc.)
____
2 What is the name of this place, if any? ______________________
3 Where is this place located? What street is it on? What is the nearest cross-street? What city is it in? What COUNTRY is it in?

On ______________________ (Street)
Near ______________________ (Cross-Street)
In____________________ (City) __________________ (State)
In ______________________ (Country)

[PLACE 3]

1 What type of a place is this? (e.g., friend's house, doctor's office, etc.) ______________________________
2 What is the name of this place, if any? ______________________
3 Where is this place located? What street is it on? What is the nearest cross-street? What city is it in? What COUNTRY is it in?

On ______________________ (Street)
Near ______________________ (Cross-Street)
In____________________ (City) __________________ (State)
In ______________________ (Country)

[PLACE 4]

1 What type of a place is this? (e.g., friend's house, doctor's office, etc.)
____
2 What is the name of this place, if any? ______________________

3 Where is this place located? What street is it on? What is the nearest cross-street? What city is it in? What COUNTRY is it in?

On ________________________ (Street)
Near ________________________ (Cross-Street)
In__________________ (City) ______________________ (State)
In ________________________ (Country)

If you wish to share information about more than four places, please let the researcher in sight know. We can provide an additional paper for you to fill out. Thank you.

If you have any comments and/or questions you would like to share, we would be happy to hear from you (Please provide comments and/or questions here):

Thank you very much for sharing your knowledge and for your honest opinions. We really appreciate your help, and your stories are very important to us. If you have any questions or concerns about the research and/or your participation, please feel free to contact Professors Aggie J. Noah, Kathy Nakagawa, and Karen J. Leong at Arizona State University. Here is their contact information:

Dr. Aggie J. Noah Aggie.Noah@asu.edu
Dr. Kathy Nakagawa nakagawa@asu.edu
Dr. Karen J. Leong Karen.Leong@asu.edu

Appendix B

Selected National AANHPI Organizations

Depending on location, you may find local ethnic-focused, Native Hawaiian, pan-Asian American, pan-Pacific Islander, and/or pan-AANHPI organizations that address matters related to AANHPIs and AANHPI women. While several feminist organizations issue policy statements and factsheets about wage gaps, sexual and gender violence, and other topics that impact AANHPI women (e.g. National Women's Law Center, Institute for Women's Policy Research, Girl's Leadership), we have chosen to highlight selected organizations that specifically address social justice at the intersections of gender, sexuality, race/ethnicity, and other systemic factors. We encourage you to seek these out.

For those that cannot locate local organizations, we list national-level organizations as resources:

Women-focused AANHPI Organizations

National Asian Pacific American Women's Forum (NAPAWF)
https://napawf.org

This national organization addresses issues of reproductive justice for Asian American, Native Hawaiian, and Pacific Islander women and girls. It particularly promotes recognition of how economic, social, and immigrant policies affect reproductive health and rights for AANPHI women, and thus engages in organizing among communities and educating about equipping community members about their rights and how to affect policies that impact bodily autonomy and sexual and reproductive health. NAPAWF provides regular fact sheets for community members to educate themselves on their Resources page.

Asian American Feminist Collective (AAFC)
https://www.asianamfeminism.org

This New York City-based group provides insightful political analyses of issues facing Asian American women that engage the intersections of gender, race, class, sexuality, citizenship, and other social factors. AAFC is explicitly queer and trans-friendly and sex- and sex worker positive. In addition, they have sought to create cross-racial coalitions with other organizations. They have produced a series of online resources that promote dialog, reflection, and action – whether online stories, zines, and online workshops and dialogs.

AAPI Women Lead https://www.imreadymovement.org

This organization seeks to bridge different generations of Asian American, Native Hawaiian, and Pacific Islander women, girls, femme, and non-binary communities in mobilizing against violence with other communities of color. They have mobilized #ImReady to address the multiple ways AANHPI women have been affected by structural violence and in 2022 initiated a "national intergenerational participatory action research (IPAR) project" about "racial and gender-based violence through a transformative justice framework", involving community-based researchers across the US, Hawaii, and Pacific Islands. The organization features online resources emphasizing storytelling and healing and wellness.

Women-focused Native Hawaiian and/or Pacific Islander Organizations

'Aha Wahine Kūhinapapa https://www.ahawahine.org

This organization serves Hawaiian women (wāhine). The website states, "'Aha Wahine Kūhinapapa now recognizes that a movement is necessary to grow the mana that can be defined, tracked, and measured to influence policy, programs and services that strengthen wāhine and families." (https://www.ahawhine.org/about)

Kalauokekahuli https://www.kalauokekahuli.org

Kalauokekahuli supports Native Hawaiian and Pacific Islander reproductive health by centering culturally-specific care and values in their prenatal, birth, and postpartum care. They provide in-person and virtual services for "Kanaka and Pasifika 'ohana" (https://www.kalauhokekahuli.org/services accessed January 20, 2024).

National NHPI Advocacy Organizations

Empowering Pacific Islander Communities (EPIC) https://empoweredpi.org

This national Native Hawaiian and Pacific Islander organization focuses on advocating social justice for NHPI families, sustaining NHPI culture, developing NHPI leaders, and promoting decolonized research that benefits NHPI communities. EPIC in particular focuses on addressing systemic barriers to health equity and access, immigration, and education.

Native Hawaiian & Pacific Islander Alliance https://www.nhpialliance.org

This alliance addresses the critical health disparities that Native Hawaiians and Pacific Islanders face. They have advocated for separate data collection for Native Hawaiian and Pacific Islanders in order to promote better health care specific to their communities.

National AANHPI Advocacy Organizations

Asian Americans Advancing Justice (AAJC) https://www.advancingjustice-aajc.org

Asian Americans Advancing Justice promotes social justice and recognition for Asian Americans by focusing on political access through voter registration, immigration rights, and census representation. It provides useful resources to educate communities about Asian American issues and recognizes the diversity across ethnic groups among the Asian American community. Importantly, even with its focus on Asian American representation, AAJC also recognizes the need to work in coalition with other ethnic/racial groups across the United States to achieve greater equity and social justice.

Asian Mental Health Collective https://www.asianmhc.org

Asian Mental Health Collective provides a variety of resources for mental health and wellness that are specific to AANHPIs. Their website provides a centralized location of information about AANHPI mental health care providers and support groups; it also has a mental health blog, a YouTube channel, and personal stories that demonstrate that mental health and emotional well-being can be discussed openly and without shame. The collective also seeks to make mental health care more accessible to Asian/Americans, Native Hawaiians, and Pacific Islanders through the Lotus Therapy Fund (information provided on website).

Asian & Pacific Islander American Health Forum (APIAHF) https://www.apiahf.org

APIAHF engages health justice for Asian Americans and Pacific Islanders in the U.S., U.S. Territories, and COFA nations. The organization's initiatives are policy oriented and do not specifically focus on women's health, but promote data disaggregation and have been particularly notable for their attention to COFA citizens' access to U.S. health care via Medicaid.

Asian Pacific Institute on Gender-Based Violence https://www.api-gb.org

Although this book did not focus on gender-based violence for reasons stated in the Introduction, gender-based violence is very much a part of AANPHI overall health. The Insitute's website provides useful information about all aspects of gender-based violence across genders and sexualities, including domestic violence, sexual violence, and trafficking. It provides resources for culturally specific advocacy, including for Muslim women and Pacific Islanders, AANHPI survivors of gender-based violence on college campuses, dating abuse and sexual assault among AANHPI teens, and resources for immigrant women workers facing sexual harassment in the work place.

Association of Asian Pacific Community Health Organizations (AAPCHO) https://aaphco.org

AAPCHO's efforts for health equity and health care quality are especially relevant to AANHPI women's sexual and reproductive health. The organization seeks to advance more culturally responsive policies among health care providers and in health care policy for AANHPI communities. The organization's many initiatives include promoting data justice, health care accessibility, and promoting the health of Pacific Islanders, and Sexual and Gender Minority patients, through training and education.

National Organization of API Ending Sexual Violence (NAPIESV) https://napiesv.org

This transnational organization emerged from an AANHPI organization in Iowa. NAPIESV focuses on Asian, Native Hawaiian, and Pacific Islander survivors of sexual violence in the U.S., U.S. Pacific territories, and Asians. In addition to supporting local and international community-based programs, it provides resources including topical written and video reports, webinars, curricula about sexual violence, healing, and transformative justice, and reading lists.

National Asian American Pacific Islander Empowerment Network (NAAPIEN) https://www.naaihmha.org

NAAPIEN also addresses mental health issues for AANHPIs. Useful resoures related to content in this book would be the "Racism and Mental Health Resources" and a much more extensive list of National AANHPI organizations than those listed here.

National Council of Asian Pacific Americans (NCAPA)
https://www.ncapaonline.org

This council consists of national AANHPI organizations, including those that are Pacific Islanders, women, Asian American, and topic specific (found on the "Member Organizations" page).

StopAAPIHATE https://stopaapihate

This organization, begun in response to increased blatant anti-Asian violence during the COVID-19 pandemic, tracks anti-AAPI hate acts and provides reports about the collected data for communities and policy makers. StopAAPIHate has inspired local organizing among Asian/American communities nationwide. The organization publishes its reports as well as the data on its website. Of specific relevance is the high rate of anti-AAPI hate acts that targeted women and elderly during the pandemic, demonstrating the ways in which gender and age are factors for hate acts due to perceived vulnerability.

Index

Pages in *italics* refer to figures and pages in **bold** refer to tables.

For Product Safety Concerns and Information please contact our EU
representative GPSR@taylorandfrancis.com
Taylor & Francis Verlag GmbH, Kaufingerstraße 24, 80331 München, Germany

www.ingramcontent.com/pod-product-compliance
Ingram Content Group UK Ltd.
Pitfield, Milton Keynes, MK11 3LW, UK
UKHW021112180425
457613UK00005B/52

* 9 7 8 1 0 3 2 5 8 3 8 6 0 *